EVERY HEALING HAS A STORY
published by Thinkaboutit Productions, Inc.
PUREBIOENERGY is a registered Trade Mark of Bioenergy Project, LLC

©2016, Zoran Hochstätter, Thinkaboutit Productions, Inc.
Photography by Zoran Hochstätter, Stephanie Coté, Hana Meglic, Gabriel Hochstätter
Book design by Ivan Pešić
Fonts used: Klinic Slab, Marco, Myriad, Sero Pro
Printed by CreateSpace, an Amazon.com Company

ISBN: 978-1522806639

Every Healing Has A Story

EXTRAORDINARY RESULTS FROM ORDINARY PEOPLE
A DIFFERENT UNDERSTANDING OF THE HEALING PROCESS

by Zoran Hochstätter

with over 100 Healing Stories
from Students, Practitioners, and Clients

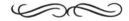

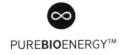

PURE**BIO**ENERGY™

Published by *Thinkaboutit Productions, Inc.* ©2016

Table of Contents

Foreword

The purpose of this book is to provoke thinking about a different way of thinking.

Many books have been written about the alternative approach to healing and many people pointed out that it isn't all that clear what is alternative, what is traditional and what was here first. It does not matter. What matters is that most of books I am talking about are trying to explain what happens during healing, what is energy, what is wrong with official medicine, science, etc.

This book is not going to explain any medical, scientific nor esoteric issues.

This book is not a recommendation for a path one should follow to achieve bliss, happiness or painless longevity.

This book is only offering a glimpse into a different worldview, into a possibility of thinking differently, having a different approach to the same problem and getting a different solution as a result of a different way of thinking.

Ten years ago, in *"Think About It"*, a Healing Documentary, I wanted to steer people towards a different, alternative way of thinking about health and healthcare. I wanted them to see that there are serious healing results possible through the use of Bioenergy. I made sure that I didn't say anything bad about anything and anybody. It is not that I shy away from a good fight but I believe, from the bottom of my heart, that there are many ways to get where we are going but there is still only one truth.

Ten years later the only thing that matters to me is that truth. I don't care so much about who does what and how they feel about themselves but I do care about the integrity of the healer and the responsibility of knowledge. It is my responsibility to do the best I can and know how. I expect it from myself and demand it from my students.

Since the information about your wellbeing is contained in the Bioenergy itself and the body knows how to use it, there is no need for any information coming from the healer. As long as the energy stays pure, it has the healing properties.

My students and I wrote this book.

I supplied the little essays about what I do and why I think everyone should learn how to heal with Purebioenergy.

My students supplied the healing stories, the results of my teaching and their learning.

They are regular people. Nothing is special about them. They come from all walks of life and all five continents. They are housewives, parents, medical doctors and nurses, nuns and pastors, retired teachers, physicists, artists, truck drivers and farmers. Many of them are chiropractors, acupuncturists, naturopaths, osteopaths, homeopaths and practitioners of many energy-healing modalities. Their education varies, literally, from the grade school to multiple PhDs.

The only thing they have in common is the fact that they attended at least one of my classes in the last eight years.

These healing stories were supplied by them, by their clients, their family members, friends and neighbors. We call them healing stories because when I read a testimonial, the whole story opens up in front of my eyes. The person is real, they have a family and friends and all of them are a part of the same story. In time of need emotions bubble up and are always present, no matter how dry the report is. They are always stories.

Some of them were sent to the therapists, my students, some of them were sent to me, some were drawings by children who were helped, some were text messages, and some were voice messages. We have hundreds and hundreds of these and the hardest was to collect and store them (thank you Stephanie) and to sift through them and edit them (thank you Cathie).

Maybe, just maybe, the message will come across that what matters is a practical application of the wisdom at hand.

Energy healing isn't worth much unless you use it. You don't have to understand it to use it and you don't even have to believe in it. It doesn't have to be explained, it has to be experienced.

So here are some healing results from people that had enough courage to use the knowledge they gained in my class. It is an inspiration to all of us, and it is a celebration of taking the self-responsibility into their hands where it belongs.

The names of clients were removed for protection of their privacy.

The names of therapists were removed for the same reason and because I did not want for this book to be an advertising campaign for anybody in particular.

This book is not litterature, I write the way I speak. My book – my rules.

Zoran Hochstätter
Siesta Key, FL April 2015

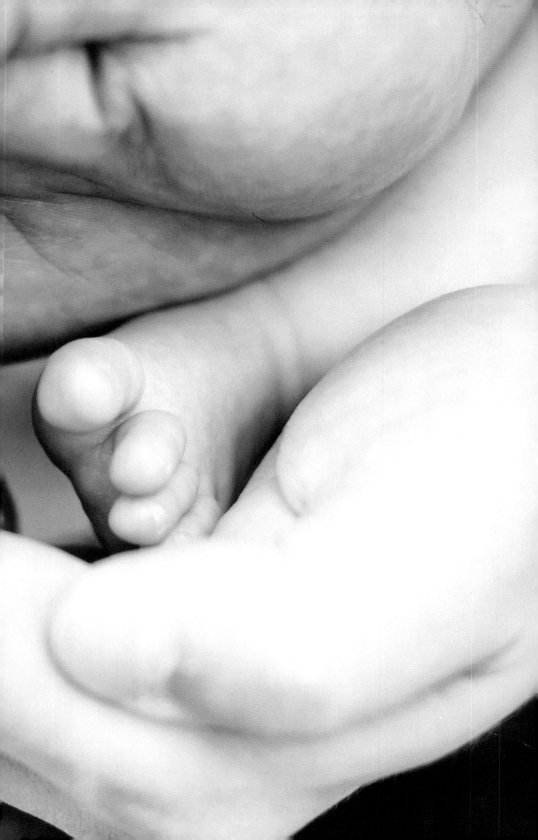

gentle

Gentle is as good a place to start as any.

Bioenergy (Bios, Greek for life) is energy of Life. It is the essential ingredient needed for you or anything else to be alive. It is gentle by definition and the harshness we sometimes observe in nature is our interpretation, a product of our conditioning.

Applying bioenergy in healing is a gentle business, especially if it is pure. There is nothing harsh in it. It is soothing and relaxing when applied properly. If it feels differently you are doing something wrong.

The information of wellbeing is streaming through the hands.

If you think life is harsh, think again. Balanced, healthy life is gentle. What makes it rough is our unhealthy attitude towards nature stemming from the cultural and social conditioning carefully nourished by the governing authorities of all civilizations for thousands of years.

The Universe, constantly growing and changing is beautiful. Being an inseparable part of nature makes us perfect, timeless.

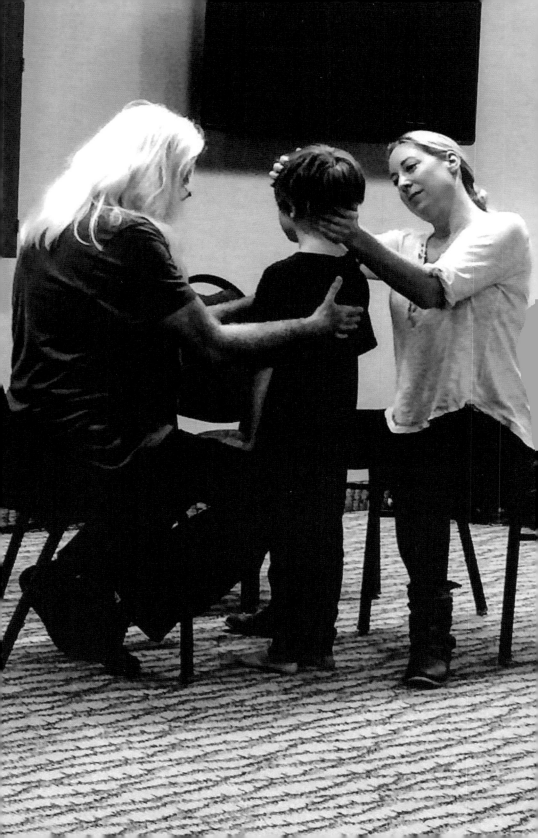

good for children

It is most upsetting for me to see sick children.

Yes, this is conditioning too. I am still, somewhat, a part of this world and am not immune to compassion the way most people understand it.

No matter what their cause and reason for being in this world is, children still need to be taken care of by adults.

The effect of Bioenergy on children is directly connected to the belief of their parents. It is their decision to expose the child to the practitioner, healer, whatever you want to call them.

Usually children react wonderfully. As long as they are not too old and not yet formed by the peer pressure, they accept the energy and their body does the rest. Everybody is happy.

Sometimes parents bring the child with emotional, psychological or mental problems and then the expectations can become much different.

When physical ailment is removed, the child walks, or poops, again we all applaud.

What happens when things are not so clean-cut? What are the expectations of parents whose children have learning disabilities or aren't showing the aptitude for being a doctor or a scientist?

When parents don't want to accept the fact that every child is capable of excelling in something, and that may be different from their wishes, then there will be disappointment in the hearts of parents.

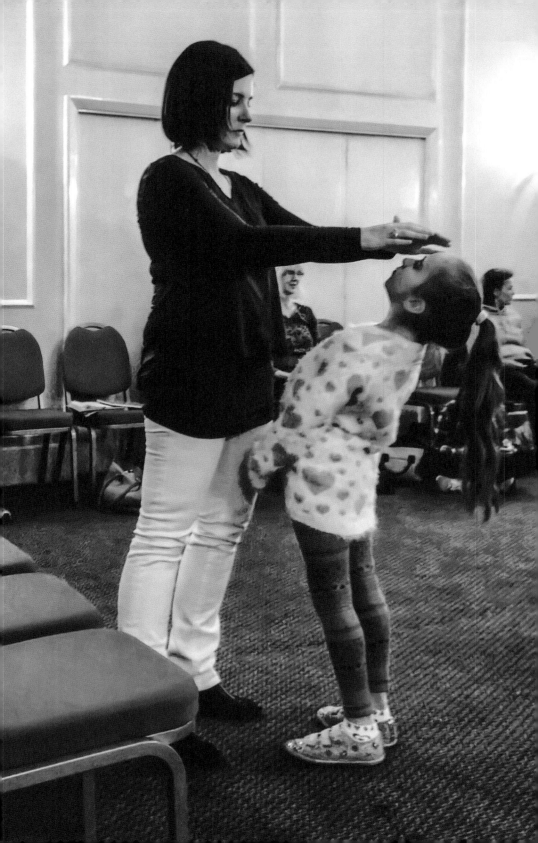

When children have problems we should work on their parents too.

Simply removing some of the stress, caused by their child's illness, helps them see their child's future in a more favorable light. Acceptance of any condition is easier. Displeasure becomes satisfaction.

Even if your children are perfectly healthy, with all their "problems", sooner or later somebody will try to convince them that they need help. Some pill or another, this supplement, or that therapy, to ease them through their growing pains.

Even you will put pressure on them to always show that little extra achievement in class or in the sports field.

Remember how it was for you and how much pressure you had from your environment. Everything was different then, of course, but nevertheless there was friction and stress.

The verbal advice clearly does not work or there wouldn't be so many "troubled" children.

Try Purebioenergy, which has all the information they need.

The toxins they get from their peers, media, school, etc. will still be there but they will cut through the crap easier.

Imagine being able to help your daughter with her hormones. Or simply prop up her own way of thinking so she does not have to be like one of those popular girls or the latest star with a perfect body and an empty head.

Maybe she won't insist for you to buy her a plastic surgery as a graduation present.

Or maybe she won't be totally disappointed and unhappy if you turn her down.

Those are big results, even though we are still talking about a healthy child.

Imagine the empowerment when you can help your child with a real medical condition. Maybe they were born with a defect. Maybe they are Autistic. Maybe they don't even have a diagnosis.

You can surely think of another hundred uses that would change your and your children's lives. Imagine how good it feels to experience that amount of self-responsibility.

Children

A Mom's DIY story.

Bioenergy makes healing an integrated part of family life.

My family first tried Bioenergy healing almost a year and a half ago and experienced deep and profound changes in our health. In just two rounds of distance therapy, my intensely immune compromised son showed clear improvement in his lab work, energy levels, and anxiety. During my sessions, my thyroid function and a fifteen years old injury in my neck improved. Encouraged by what we experienced, I went to learn to do this therapy myself. A year later, our health is better than it has been over the course of my son's entire short life and mine is better than when I was a child.

Learning to provide this form of pure energy therapy for my own family, and later for other families, changed how we think about health and illness. We feel empowered to help our bodies heal in the face of everything from serious diseases like cancer or autoimmune conditions, to the more average illnesses of childhood like measles or whooping cough.

Any family that learns this method has the potential to experience deep and lasting changes in their health.

Our Health Keeps Improving.

In the year of providing this therapy to my own family, and receiving it myself, we keep seeing improvements in our health. My son's health issues all revolved around his severely compromised immune system, massive gut inflammation, serious and moderate food allergies, and bouts of lost coordination that caused him to stagger sideways when he ran. Anxiety, low physical stamina, and borderline anemia were some of his lesser issues.

For the first 18 months of his life, we had seen a number of specialists who told us to expect a lifetime of regular antibiotics, probably overall worsening of his health, and lingering illnesses. Even after working with doctors who understood his issues, the best we had attained was a fragile kind of stability easily set back by a new food, cold, or even the normal stresses of a toddler.

After learning Bioenergy Healing and providing therapy whenever he seemed to need it, he is now within the normal range on all of his blood test results, has the same stamina as any other preschooler, and can catch a cold and recover without issue. Shrimp and peanut allergies are gone, other allergy reactions are reduced, and he hasn't lost coordination since the first round of therapy.

My own health improved so much I no longer need any medication for my thyroid, allergies, or asthma. For the first time since grade school, I can leave my house without an inhaler for my asthma.

Real help for illness and disease — provided at home.

In our journey to find health for my son, we never settled for the prognosis we were given. We tried many different means to improve his health, from medicine to supplements to homeopathy. Each of those steps contributed to our understanding of his issues and helped us achieve our first taste of stability. But what we experienced in our first two rounds of Bioenergy therapy was greater than anything we had tried to date. My ability to provide the therapy whenever he needed it has been instrumental in the progress he has made.

As I work with other families experiencing improvement with this therapy, I often remind them of how easy it is to learn such a powerful and unique way to support the health of their families.

Parents providing this simple treatment themselves allow children with autism, allergies, asthma, or anyone with any other health issue to be able to get therapy easily around their school and work schedules, making healing an integrated part of their lives at home.

Therapists also receive benefit with each round of therapy they perform as it boosts their immune system, as well. Our family feels capable and ready to address complex health issues by supporting the body's most knowledgeable healer – the immune system. Anyone who is interested in regaining control of their family's health would benefit from learning PureBioenergy™ healing.

This Mom learned bioenergy healing from Zoran Hochstätter and is now a certified PureBioenergy™ therapist.

4 years old boy - serious progress — therapist's report

The 4 yrs. old boy I was working on showed some serious progress, the first day he wouldn't sit too much and finally he would sit with his mom and get the treatment but not really sitting still. By the 4th day he pushed away mom and dad and sat by himself and received the whole treatment being extremely compliant with everything I asked him to do. He also wanted to help me give the treatments to other people and was warming their hearts while I was warming their heads. He was very engaged and interested in what was happening in the room with the therapy by day 3 & 4 - which is quite a turn around from day 1-2.

9 years old boy has limited us of his legs due to spinal issues prior to birth.

Spinal column never closed around the spinal cord in certain parts of the spine. He has no use of legs, cannot control bowel movement nor the bladder. His legs cannot carry his body's weight.

"I realize that it has only been one week but wanted to give you an update on S. His back is definitely stronger. He is able to sit stronger and longer without having to use his hands to steady himself. There are more muscles firing in his legs along with more movements in both legs. His left ankle and toes are also moving more than ever before. He seems to have more awareness and feeling in his legs as well. Cognitively, he is more settled and seems more grounded. He doesn't seem to get as easily upset about things.

We went camping this weekend and we went swimming as a family at the campground. As soon as S. got into the water, I could see the differences in him. He was so much stronger and was doing an actual butterfly stroke to swim between people and to get toys we were throwing back and forth. The changes are exciting and I look forward to each new change!"

A skeptical mom

"My name is Amanda and I can tell you from personal experience Energywork has had a positive effect on my life and more importantly, my Child's life. You see, as a mother who leans more towards

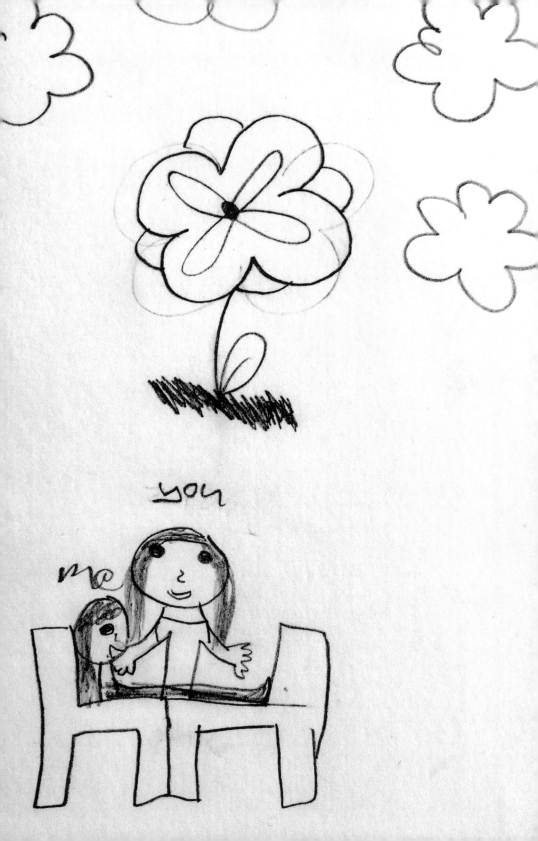

scientific explanations of life was a little skeptical of Reiki & Bioenergy as anything more than a placebo effect. ... At three my son was not only used to having to take anti-inflammatory medicine constantly but was also on prescription allergy medicine that he had to take every single day and it wasn't helping. ... I finally figured why not and talked to one of my teachers about what she does with Bioenergy work and how it could help my son. My son first saw her in December the session took about 20 minutes, which is a lot less time then you'll ever spend waiting in a Dr.'s office, and I noticed soon after that he was sleeping a lot better. Since then we have had Bioenergy work done for my son on a regular basis and now he no longer has to take a pill every day, he sleeps through the night without coughing, and even when he does get really sick, and he has, it's no where near as bad as it was and he can actually sleep and get better, instead of staying up every night miserable. So I say this, from someone who definitely didn't think there was any validity in this "hippie mumbo jumbo", I know it has helped my child and I'm truly glad to have met a Bioenergy therapist and am just utterly grateful for all the help she has given my son."

Autism – daughter

The day we, (my mother in law and I) came home from Level One course in Sarasota, we did Bioenergy healing on my husband. My daughter showed interest in what we were doing. She has a language impairment and was diagnosed with that, for a lack of a better diagnosis, since everybody who has seen her says that she shows slight signs of every condition you can imagine, like ADD, Autism, Social Anxiety, etc.

She later asked me to "fix" her foot, she has a nasty foot corn, but I was more interested in helping with her Autistic signs and her fears. We quickly started the first session and she was laughing hard because she said I was tickling her feet. It was right away that we noticed her to be connecting in a way we had not seen before. She showed big changes, she seemed more alert and attentive to our actions. The biggest thing about these changes is that they happened all of a sudden and they have stayed. She seems to be growing into more of a little human being. She listens better and understands more what she is asked to do. She is braver now and can play outside and go around the block riding her bicycle, which she would never do before. We are really excited to see my daughter blooming!!!

Since then, I have done 4 sessions on her and she seems to enjoy every second of it. Teachers only have had very nice things to say about her, they are really happy with whatever happened, they say she seems more alert, more willing to work, and best of all, she has been recognizing when she needs to ask for help and she is actually doing it. They've also told me that on a few occasions she actually helped classmates who were struggling with their work, something she had never done before.

By the way, the whole time during the level I training, I was regretting not having her with us but I really believe she was with us and started her transformation then.

All I have to say is that it worked on my daughter and I thank Grammy (my mother in Law) for giving me the best present I had ever and I will ever receive.

Thank you Grammy and thank you Zoran.

Autism on my 3 years old grandson

After repeating Levels 1 & 2 in Manhattan Beach in January, I have been doing Bioenergy on my family on a weekly basis. I did the Autism protocol for 2 full 4- days sessions, a few weeks apart. Everyone noticed the change in my little grandson. My daughter, friends & his teachers said he was much more verbal. All of a sudden, I noticed he was making better eye contact with me. It was so exciting to see him make so much progress - in such short time. I certainly will continue doing Bioenergy on him on a regular basis.

Autism "Instant improvement" – parents' feedback

"S. (8 yrs.) LOVED the therapy! He was very aware of the energy and excited that it would help some of his issues. I didn't notice results the first few days but I did the following week. His usual dread for homework disappeared and was replaced with positive eagerness to complete. He was motivated to start a new wii U exercise program that focuses on balance and core strength and has done really well with it. His speech and occupational therapist have come to talk to me each separately on his "instant improvement" with balance, self-esteem, and speech. It's been exciting to see him improve so quickly! We have taken him off almost all his medication for sleeping, he no longer takes allergy pills or sprays, nor does he take any acid reflux medications. He sleeps great now with no night terrors. We are very excited about his progress and can't wait for the next sessions!!"

Autism - "when you're happy and you know it" - better sleep, eye contact, more sociable - M's granddaughter

I would like to share my experience with my 3 years old granddaughter which has been truly remarkable! I observed incredible changes beginning after the first session. One of the most noteworthy effects was a change in her sleeping patterns. Normally she would go to bed about 12 pm and was up by 4 or 4:30 every morning. After the first session, she slept until almost 8am the next morning. Since then, she has become habitual at retiring about 10 and waking up about 7:30. (My pregnant daughter is delighted with more sleep herself too!) Another big change we noticed from the second day of therapy is making eye contact. She virtually never did this! And now she will look at each one of us and the length of time she looks at us is increasing all the time. She has become much more verbal since therapy, and in fact, managed to make a sound for each letter of the whole alphabet about 2 weeks after the therapy finished. Before that she only attempted sounds for about 6 or 7 letters. She is also trying to repeat many more words. Her attention span in most everything seems to have increased and a few days ago we got through the WHOLE song of "If you're happy and you know it clap your hands..." AND she clapped and stamped too! This was delightful for my whole family! It has been totally exciting indeed.

An update on my granddaughter after completion of a second treatment.

Her second session was done remotely and I was delighted when I returned home and saw her more verbal, more attentive, more social, more everything! But the BEST thing so far (and things just keep getting better and better!!) was yesterday when she took my hand and my daughter's hand and said "come" so clearly and with intention as she led us into another room and tried to make us sit on the floor with her to play letters. This is the very first time EVER she has participated in a speaking/action activity! The other major noteworthy point is that she is so much more social now. She AL-MOST NEVER interacted with (or even looked at) anyone before we started Bioenergy Therapy and now it seems like she actually prefers being in the company of us (we are a very large, noisy family) than being only in her own world. Wow! How about that?

I continue to be amazed and dazzled by the changes in her.

Autistic 3 years old - Therapist's result

A woman brought her Autistic 3 year old son to me.

She warned me that he would not sit still because he was too hyper-active. I assured her that I would not attempt to restrain him, but I would work "with" him while he sat on her lap.

When they returned the next day for his 2nd session, his mother said that the boy's father came by the night before to give his son a haircut. She said that, normally, he simply would not sit still and squirm all over the place, making it quite difficult to cut his hair. "Instead", she said, "he sat there the whole time like a little man."

She added that, while at pre-school that afternoon (before his 2nd session), he was able to carry his own lunch tray from the cafeteria line to his table, something he had never done before.

Bioenergy Healing Helps Children with PANDAS/PANS

A therapist's experience

Over the course of the past year, I have provided Purebioenergy™ healing for a growing number of children with a PANS or PANDAS diagnosis. Bioenergy healing provides real relief to children and their families during flare ups of the condition, as well as afterwards when they want to take further steps to improve their child's overall immune system. Since the method works by addressing the overall health of the client, working with children having an active PANS flare has a lasting impact on their immune system even after the flare is over.

What is PANS or PANDAS?

Both acronyms describe a neuropsychiatric condition that comes on suddenly and severely in children. Some research indicates that exposure to strep or other infections can make a child susceptible or actually trigger a flare, but the understanding of PANS is still evolving. Typically, parents describe a flare as one or all of the following:

- Tics – vocal or physical

- Intense anxiety and fears

- Severe OCD

- Total loss of appetite

- Rapid mood swings

- Bed-wetting

- Temper tantrums or rages

- Fatigue

- Sometimes bodily pain like swollen glands, headaches, gut pain, or back pain

Often treated with antibiotics, families tell me the drugs seem to provide less relief each time. Their focus then shifts to avoiding future flares, but since the exact triggers are unknown and can vary from child to child, avoiding all possible triggers becomes extremely life limiting.

Families want REAL HEALING

The families I work with are looking for something more. Real healing for their children. Stronger (optimized) immune systems to manage any triggering events. Normal childhoods.

They turn to Purebioenergy to help boost their child's immune system and then find so much more than that in terms of stopping flares, reducing their intensity, and slowing down how quickly they come on.

Using PUREBIOENERGY™ healing

I provide therapy based on set protocols, addressing the issues specific to each child. Therapy takes place one time per day, usually for 20 minutes, over 4 consecutive days. The therapy then builds in strength for another 8 to 10 days.

During the full course of therapy, families see improvements:

- Children are typically calmer after each day's therapy, which is very different than the usual path of a flare
- Mood improves rapidly
- Body aches or issues usually start decreasing within the first 2 sessions of the 4 days treatment, often showing a reduction on the first day.
- OCD and anxiety start decreasing rapidly
- Vocal tics usually decrease rapidly by the 2nd session of the 4 days treatment
- Physical stamina usually increases
- Old infections sometimes come to the surface during therapy and seem to finally resolve. MRSA (drug resistant staph) or strep are frequent ones that appear and resolve very quickly over the course of therapy.

With strong results during flares, families often choose to have additional rounds of therapy. With each round of therapy, improvements grow stronger and last longer.   Parents have noted that after the first or second full course of therapy, flares seem to come on less often or more slowly, which allows them time to schedule therapy before things become overwhelming.

For those children who have a chronic level of OCD, their symptoms outside of the flare also decrease with each round of treatment.   Most importantly, they report that the times between flares are happier and smoother for the child and the whole family.

Families also choose Bioenergy Healing for other health issues.

For the families who see such improvement during a flare, it's an easy choice to do additional rounds of therapy for other health issues.   Their children often also have allergies, asthma, or other health concerns that can directly benefit from Purebioenergy even as their overall immune system is being balanced and optimized again and again.

This method of therapy is pure Bio energy. (Life itself)

Purebioenergy™ is unique even amongst other forms of energy

work in that it only ever focuses on the health of the client, not their illness. The energy we work with is the same intelligent energy that surrounds us all the time. It works as well at a distance as it does in person. For families whose children are not able to travel to a therapist or group clinic, that's a huge benefit. Children, unlike adults, usually don't have many preconceived notions about what kinds of therapy will work. They simply want to feel better and quite honestly tell you whether they do or not.

For parents who have seen their children undergo swift and severe changes in personality during a PANS flare, this therapy is easy to evaluate.

The improvements in their children tell parents everything they need to know.

Boy with Tick

… "We came to see you about couple of months ago regarding my son's ticks and stomach. I wanted to give you an update on how we are doing…

My son's tick is gone. I have not seen it at all for probably 2 weeks. It gradually decreased and then for two weeks or so I have not seen it at all so far…. I would like to mention that it took longer then two weeks to see the results, but the results are truly amazing…

Everyday, I thank God for sending me to you. I'm soooo happy that his tick has been reduced to minimum and (possibly it is totally gone)…. Thank you again."

Three months later…not a single tick!

Six months later…family reported that he still hasn't had any more!

Children's headaches and earaches gone with the help of Bioenergy

Since attending my level 1 course, I have enjoyed working on my kids to give them immediate relief from pain and discomfort. I have been able to completely alleviate my son's headaches in just one session. I have been able to help my daughter with clogged ears/ear congestion, and she reported hearing a "crackling" noise in her ear as I did the ear protocol.

One particular example stands out in my mind - one night my son was suffering from ear pain. I had tried a number of things to help him, including elevating his head on pillows, giving him a hot water bottle and even a hot onion compress, but I did not want to give him medication if I could avoid it. When he woke up for the third time in the middle of the night, crying from pain, I decided do bio energy. He went from crying at the beginning of the session, to reporting that his ear pain was completely gone and he was ready to go back to sleep, at the end of the session 15 minutes later. After that, he stayed asleep all night, and was much better the next day.

I recently had a similar experience with my daughter, who woke up crying with ear pain. This time around, I skipped the hot compresses, and just did bioenergy right off the bat. Her pain was gone and she slept soundly through the night.

Although I got trained in bioenergy for my son's autism - which we continue to treat him for, and he is improving - although it is a longer process - it has been very encouraging to see both kids improve so rapidly and markedly through bioenergy treatments, and I have discovered a new kind of health-enhancing first-aid which I can offer to comfort them at any time.

Cyst behind the Ear - surgery not needed

Around Christmas, my daughter discovered my 3 years old grandson had a bump behind his left ear. She took him to the Pediatrician who referred him to a Surgeon. The Surgeon wanted to operate right away, but my daughter wanted to wait. When she told me about it, I did 2 rounds of Bioenergy on him using the Tumor Protocol.

About 6 weeks later, she took him back to the Pediatrician for a regular check up. The Pediatrician said that the cyst appeared smaller & he didn't need surgery at this time. I was so excited when my daughter told me this that I did another round of Bioenergy (total of 3). And I will continue to use Bioenergy on him until his cyst completely goes away.

Who needs a Surgeon?

Dyslexia

I have been treating a 7 years old boy for what his mother thinks is Dyslexia.

He switches letters and numbers around.

Anyway, I have completed 3 rounds of 5 consecutive days with him and have just started my 4th. He really likes it - for reasons he cannot seem to pinpoint. I have been doing the ADD protocol on him.

Since I began these treatments, he has improved on his spelling tests, and his Spanish and piano teachers say he has been performing much better. He has also begun to take initiative and has started to sleep in his own bed.

From a mother of a child with autism

"I noticed that after the November healing my daughter was having better bowel movements, she was receptive and more willing to try different foods which was a great improvement. I also noticed she was more appropriate with her speech and behavior. I felt she was more focused during homeschooling. Overall she had a very noticeable change. Thank you so much for that."

An email from a Mom of an autistic son

"Teacher says he is solving problems now through logic more and more, trying to find solutions, he doesn't just copy anymore. Also non functioning intestines working now again, night vision completely returned,... He doesn't need glasses anymore.

Hip inflammation gone - back playing soccer

"My friend's nephew had a hip inflammation (first left then right). The parents had him see all kinds of doctors (specialists), perform tests.... and could not find an explanation or a reason for the inflammation and a terrible pain that he was in. Doctors tried to treat him with steroids, but it helped only little while taking them, then the pain returned. After the second day of treatment of Bioenergy he went to soccer practice, and was able to play and do all the drills with no discomfort. He is now pain free, getting better and better in soccer, and his father tells me that he became more confident. At the same time he used to have occasional stomach pains..... He had no more stomach problems since the treatment."

Doctors do not know what the diagnosis is but appears like neuromuscular condition – the child cannot talk, hear and has a lack of motor skills.

Mother's report

"My daughter's speech therapist stopped me the other day in school and was all excited about how she cooperated with her for 45 minutes. She answered everything correctly (pointed to pictures) and even said a word. Her agitation was gone a week after your treatment, as well."

I am noticing that B. is becoming more communicative and she expresses her needs on her own, without being asked what she wants. I have a feeling she wants to speak and uses new sounds for it. If I show her how to do something and tell her that she should look there, not at me, she listens and then actually does what I ask her to do (simple things, to be sure). Small changes but very positive never the less. First I want to tell you that we are noticing further small, but frequent changes. Bogdana, her riding therapist, notes the following changes: riding facing backwards she no longer shakes like she used to, she has a nice posture and sits comfortably on a horse without a saddle. She swims faster and further than before. She started playing with the ball again and she jumps around in the water, which she didn't do for a long time.She is generally more active and expresses herself much more spontaneously."

Young Child

For the first time, this evening, I worked with a young boy aged 3. It was the MOST amazing experience with him! He was SO excited to sit and let me "do my thing" He REALLY liked the part at the end, smiling at his mom and me. I was so surprised at his willingness to sit and let me warm his head and heart with very little fidgeting. During the session, he said, "Mommy, I think she's trying to get my cough to come out...." in the most excited voice you could imagine. After we finished up and mom was getting him situated in the car, she turns to me and said, "He really enjoyed that! He's already asking when we are coming back!"

LOOK
AT
THIS

THOUGHTS ABOUT BIOENERGY

THE OLD SAGES and scientists called it Chi, Ki, Prana, Bioplasma, Orgon, Aether, Zero Point Field, Bioenergy, or whatever they called the life sustaining force of the Universe, which is more of a concept than a physical fact in the sense of classical physics. Something we cannot see but can certainly feel, see and measure its effects.

BIOENERGY doesn't have a set frequency in the way Mr. Hertz defined it and is understood in Newtonian physics. It is rather an interference of many frequencies combined with some other events (movements) in the Universe. This "new", still, frequency is the information necessary for us to be alive and healthy. It is inseparable part of nature, it is not mechanical and we cannot make a machine that produces it.

Five things you must do to become a change you want to see in the world

1.

You must invest time. You must observe masters of a certain modality and see their results, over and over.

2.

You must invest money. The mountain will not come to you. You have to go to the mountain.

3.

In choosing the healing modality you must listen to your intuition, to your heart. If it doesn't resonate with you, drop it.

4.

You must not be a miser. If you invested money in wrong training it doesn't mean you lost that money. It was money well spent on finding the right way.

5.

Any guru can show you a path but you must walk it yourself. (Room and board not included).

Let me explain >>>

1.

Nobody can become a master in a month, a year, or two. Most of the knowledge needed to master your work in the "working/learning" methods, like the Purebioenergy®, comes from practice. "Working/learning" method means that, after you are familiar with the theory, the rest of knowledge is acquired by and through working. The knowledge is contained in the energy itself.

When you practice the healing without any additives, be it cultural, social or medical, you are also exposed to the effects of pure Bioenergy. The same energy that reaches the client, the energy causing the transformation of the way they think and act, flows through you. If you remove yourself from the healing process, you will eventually, slowly, go through the same process.

Enjoy the learning process, the work. Enjoying the learning makes you grow. Impatience, hurrying to become a master because you will then make a lot of money, will backfire. There are many other honorable ways to make a lot of money fast.

2.

A good teacher will not come to you since, after all, you live in East Podunk on a limited income and you cannot travel. Or maybe you live in NYC and you expect that everything must come to you.

It is true that when you are ready the teacher will appear, but not at your doorstep. Teacher appearing means that you are now aware of him, or her, and it is up to you to ask for teaching. The ill person in need of healing has to come to a healer so that the flow of energy is moving in the right direction. Healing, as a part of the Universe, follows the universal rules of nature and it is the more coherent potential that is going to ensure the right direction of the energy flow. A good teacher of an energy healing method does much more than to show and explain the craft of the techniques used in the modality. The knowledge he teaches is also contained in the energy we use, so the flow of energy has to be carefully controlled and guided in teaching as well.

3.

How will you choose the method to use? How will you know if it is a good method? Will you believe their advertising? You will have to try it and see. You won't know until you see the results.

If you follow the marketing you will eat at McDonalds and drink Coca Cola. Is that the best we can do in nutrition?

Which healing modality is the most "in your face"? Is it the best? (A hint, it changes every few months, depending what's on Oprah).

When you spend enough money on marketing you can sell anything. Why is that? That's because we don't think with our own head. We think with somebody else's head. And when we compare what we learned about different healing methods, and their results, we have to be careful not to judge them with different criteria. Don't feel that you have to use knowledge you paid for even if you see that it is inferior to the method you learned after that.

4.

Whenever you learn something new, you are investing in yourself.

Don't be a miser. Do you crave real knowledge or just a piece of paper, the ever-popular Certificate? A Certificate from a trustworthy person will separate you from the beginners and Sunday healers. Find somebody you trust; trust their knowledge because you have seen their results, not because they tell you they are great. You will then have to practice seriously for a while, a year or two, to get enough experience to know if you like the modality in the first place and if you want to give it all your attention.

If you realize that the healing method wasn't right for you, you should rejoice. Now you know something. You've learned. All the time and money was not lost. It was a necessary part of the journey to find the truth.

What is the value of the truth?

5.

A teacher can tell you what you have to do to get results. And then you have to do it. Studying Buddhism does not make you a Buddhist. To be a Buddhist you have to practice Buddhism. Practicing Buddhism means you cannot take a little part you liked in Catholicism, a little Islam, a part of Taoism, and whatever else seems cool.

Of course you can take whatever you want and mix it all up. There is no law against it. You can start your own church and save on taxes too. In healing sometimes people do things like that and their results suffer. How long has a certain method been around? Are there many documented cases? Browsing through what's offered on the market today is just that, browsing. You browse so you can see what is out there.

After you buy it you have to use it. YOU have to walk the talk. (Now return to 1.)

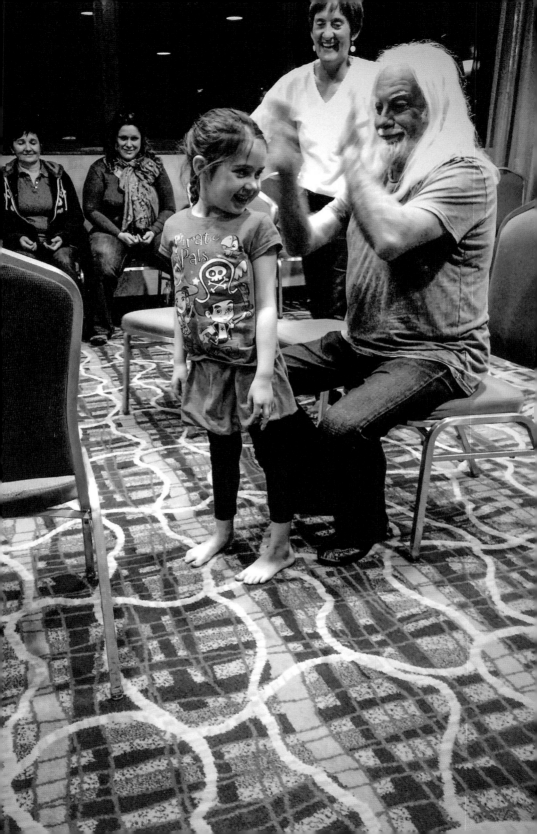

makes me feel good!

Every time I work with Purebioenergy I am invigorated.

Supplying somebody with Bioenergy is a relatively simple procedure. I channel it; I am a vessel for it as it passes through me on the way to the other body. In the process, though, all of it passes through me. Think of all the information of wellbeing, health, happiness, life itself that flows through my hands and my eyes.

Why shouldn't that have an effect on me as well? It does, of course, and the effect manifests as calm content. I am full of energy but not agitated.

It makes me feel good physically but I'm also satisfied emotionally because I helped somebody and for that I am grateful.

Gratitude is good.

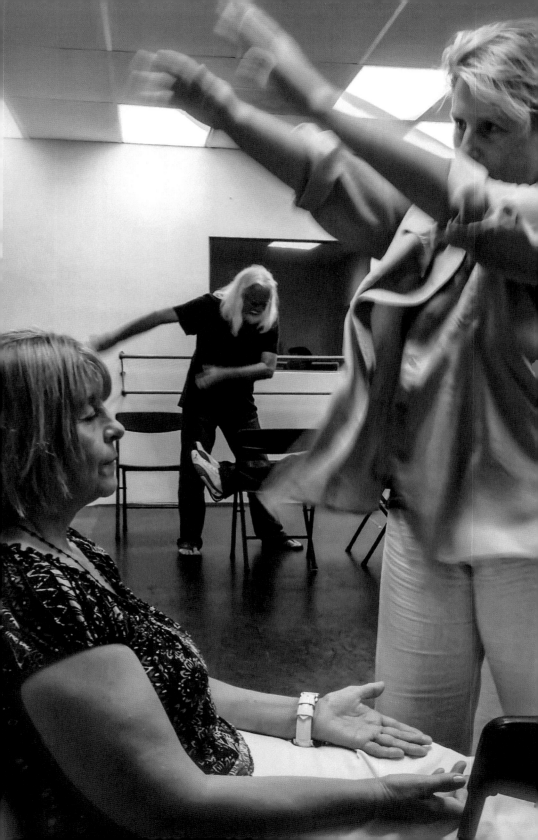

noninvasive

During therapy all that enters the body and mind is information of wellbeing. There is no invasion in any other way. Information entering your mind and body contains no negative elements like fear, anger, hate, pity, sorrow and concern. All those are our conditioning and our own interpretation of compassion. In correct application of (pure) Bioenergy the one that applies it should be removed from the process of healing. He or she is a channel, a simple conduit for the pure Bioenergy on its way to the subliminal level of the patient's mind where it will cause the transformation of the way they think and act, resulting in healing on all levels.

One has to remember that only the correct use of Bioenergy will not be invasive. Bioenergy, Chi, Prana, Zero Point Field, Divine, or whatever you want to call it, is creative thought energy. If our ego talks us into thinking that we, with our heavily conditioned minds, can add something to the process with everything we learned in school, at home, in church or on a weekend course, we are a walking proof that we did not understand how energy works.

When, in healing, we offer our own understanding and interpretation of somebody's problem and the solution for it, we are being highly invasive. We penetrate other persons mind with our beliefs or adopted worldview and are by that no different than media, government, church, whatever.

Some users (healers) know that they should remove themselves from the healing process and most of them don't. Some know they should exclude their ego but what is your ego but your mind. As long as your mind is involved in the healing process, your ego is guiding you. And not just you; you are pushing your whole self on them.

Invasive isn't only poking into the body with sharp, or blunt, objects. When you force your thoughts and ideas onto people you are being invasive as well.

The information needed for healing is already contained in the Bioenergy. Period.

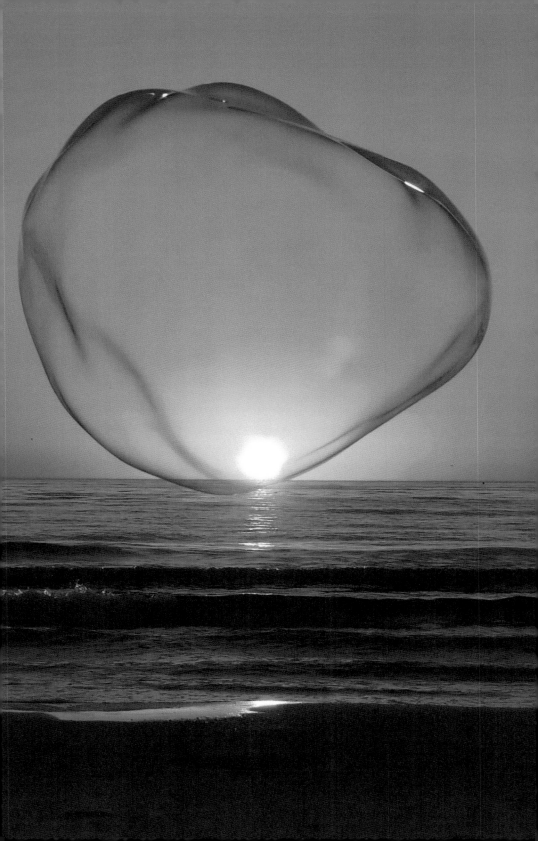

THOUGHTS ABOUT BIOENERGY

THERE ARE MANY FREQUENCIES we cannot see or feel, yet we know of their existence, and we use them on daily basis. Think of TV, radio, radar, cell phone and many others. Most of us really don't understand how a DVD player works but that does not prevent us from using it. We enjoy those films and do not wonder whether Sean Connery is really in that box and how he got in.

WHY THEN, are we so reluctant using the benefits of Bioenergy for restoring our health? Why do we think we need to know how this works?

BECAUSE WE WERE TAUGHT what to believe, what is important and what is not. And we were taught that only an approved, scientifically correct way of thinking makes anything possible.

THINK HARDER, Earth was round before we knew it and sun comes up without your doctor's approval. (And it happens pretty much every morning.)

Practitioners and Students

Immediate results after Level One What a joy!

I am Italian and I have just finished the Level 1 seminar in London.

I treated about twenty people with really great results.

In particular, people with back problems, herpes, anxiety and stress, labyrinthitis and stomach problems. In all these cases a cycle was sufficient to solve the problem. The people were really shocked and I myself, considering I started a little over a month ago.... My mother in particular, who was suffering from asthmatic bronchitis, from the second day of treatment had a marked improvement. The fourth day was fully restored. What a joy!

Switched over to this method - student gets own healing during seminar - Vancouver seminar review

Thank you so much for a truly fabulous seminar and weekend. I have been practicing Bio-Energy for the past 3 years and have switched over to this method completely right away. I feel confident using this Method and love it's simplicity and effectiveness.

The last day of the course towards the end of the day I felt so amazing. I was infused with ......well it can only be described as bliss. My ankles which had been bothering me again (arthritis) have been completely better since the seminar.

Doing therapy on others and Groups

Doing Purebioenergy healing on others has been a greater gift to me than I could ever imagine, especially being able to so quickly help my friends and family to return to a state of total health. Seeing the ones you love struggle for so long with health conditions and discomfort, and then being able to help them in a real way to experience a brand new way of being totally pain free, ignites such a feeling of service and love that is better than anything I've ever known. Most of all, I feel honored and humbled to even have the knowledge to be able to dedicate time to the wellness of others. Purebioenergy Healing is a gift to this planet and all living things.

Empowered and excited

"I am practicing as a therapist on a full time basis with amazing results, clients returning month after month. This has truly changed my whole life. No more lupus no more arthritis, no more depression. Only a bright happy future, which is rubbing off, on everyone around me.

I am not sure other than the birth of my children, I have ever been this empowered or excited about a form of healing. To literally move another human body, "without touching them" is one of the most amazing things I have ever encountered. What a privilege that I have been guided to this form of healing that will one day change healing as we have known it."

Experience as patient and student

Today is Canadian Thanksgiving. All day I've been thinking of the things I have to be grateful for this year. Aside from family and friends the single most important thing that happened to me was being introduced to this method. I got to experience it as a patient and a student. It has transformed injury and pain into the greatest opportunity to help others. Plus my arm and shoulder are functioning again. Oh...and my feet are tingling. Can't wait to be ready for level two!

Thank you so much!

FIBROID GONE - Client Astonished

I treated a woman (in a small group clinic) for a protruding fibroid tumor and this is what she had to say about her tumor disappearing after Day 1 of bioenergy treatment:

"It is flipping amazing, but when I am laying down on my back, I cannot feel the lump. I have felt it for over 2 years now, maybe longer. In the last year it is very pronounced. I don't mean sometimes I feel it, I can always feel it, and I am pressing down deep into my belly and there is no lump. This is astonishing."

Good feedback since Level II - results speak for themselves

I got news last weekend that a lady I worked on with a heart condition - she would feel dizzy every few hours - and who I worked on last Oct has dramatically improved and did so since the date of the 1st session.

I also worked Distance Healing on my wife who had a slipped disk in her back last month and she is much improved and has surprised everyone, including me, with the speed of recovery.

Last week worked on a suspected fractured rib and the guy told me that the pain went immediately after the 1st day. I only got to do 2 sessions but he was back doing Thai Boxing the following week. I think I actually scared off the boxer guy - he had 2 friends present when I worked and I had them sit in the healing position and they were surprised when they felt pins and needles and heat in their hands.

I also worked Long Distance on a cat that had suspected kidney failure - there was healing crisis - the cat is fine now as verified by the vet. So, I am getting very good feedback since level 2 and more so with the distance work. I really have no doubts now about Bioenergy; the results speak for themselves!!!

Healing Everything / Level One student from Maine

I really don't even know where to begin with this story, but boy is it a story! I have witnessed, and or, experienced Bioenergy treatment healing so many diseases that it fills me with such depth of gratitude beyond anything I have ever known. I have seen burns healed, movement restored, PTSD, Anxiety, Panic attacks, Depression, suicidal thoughts, brain fog, fatigue, joint, neck, heel, shoulder, kidney, chest, hip, herpes and back pain GONE!!!!!!! I am witnessing someone's hearing being restored! I'm sure there's more but I just cannot think of it all, and it has only just begun for me!!!!!!

How healing can be very useful even if it does not cure the illness

My father was diagnosed with stage 4 (terminal) lung cancer, which had already spread to his bones and spine, and was given a couple of months to live. After discussing the case with Zoran, we concluded that it was too late to apply the tumor protocol, but it was possible to ease my father's breathing and to manage his pain. I then applied a quick warm-and-clean protocol to his lungs 5 to 10 times a day, working at a distance (he was in hospital while I was home). He reported that his breathing improved for a while after each Bioenergy session! My father passed away about a month after receiving his diagnosis. He didn't need a single painkiller during that time, unlike many who suffer a great deal during the last stage of cancer. I am grateful that I was able to make my father's life more bearable during those difficult last days.

How happy these people became/Results after Level 1

In the last two weeks I have seen 10 people, two of which I am waiting for feedback. The other eight produced amazing results, which include:

Sciatica - gone after first session

Neck pain and migraine - gone after second session

Broken back - after the second session the patient was able to cook dinner for her family, which was the first time in 18 months since breaking her back in two places

Fused spine - patient now feels less pain and can sleep till 7am, previously waking up every day at 3 or 4 am

Sore back - pain gone and patient has lost feelings of depression

Depression - gone and patient feels great

Bladder problem - gone

Arthritis – patient's fingers were curled and hands shook. Now shaking almost gone with more movement in fingers

The big thing was how happy these people became during the

treatments. Being healthier had an amazing effect on their quality of life and happiness. It was great and I so looked forward to seeing them for their next session to see what new exciting changes had taken place. Love this stuff, its great.

Review from Holistic Health Practitioner

Since taking this Bio-Energy course I have worked on a number of people. The results have been nothing short of miraculous. People I work on are absolutely shocked when after just 10 minutes of working on them their pain is completely eliminated. It is so wonderful to be able to help people in this way. I have been in the healing field for over 8 years and never have I done so much in so little time. This method is truly miraculous in nature. It defies what we presently understand about life. This energy field we live in, and are supported by, truly can be used to heal ourselves, and those we love. Thanks so much for inviting me to this training and for your continued support as I spread my wings and become an even more effective healer.

Working on her family

The visit with my family on my recent trip to NY was yet another undeniable proof and reinforcement of how powerful and immediate the method of Purebioenergy Healing is. I had multiple opportunities to help my family and loved ones - my sisters, my nephew, my mom, etc. - with immediate results... even when I performed just an abbreviated and focused healing treatment for them.

Even though I have witnessed and experienced countless examples of this since I have become a practitioner, each new instance still fills me with wonder and gratitude. And when the person you are helping is someone you love and care about, the ability to bring them immediate relief and healing is an immeasurable soul-filling blessing.

Insights and results over the years, all levels

It's hard to list the top results of any Level of practicing. Every little change is a big result in my eyes but sometimes patients comment on massive changes as "nothing has changed" for them, which could well mean that their body has accepted the information of health just like that and they cannot remember it having been any different!

Results that have left the biggest impact for me, are those where the healing of a client changed family life as a whole. One of my first ever patients suffering from Non-Hodgkin's Lymphoma was given months to live and after his first ever treatment his wife called me, in tears, saying that he had left the house willingly for the first time in over 2 years, talking their dog for a walk …. 4 months later he got the all clear and went for a motorcycle tour in Greece, he was dreaming about that for 10 years …

Other experiences include cancer to vanish within a 4 day treatment on a few occasions, scoliosis correcting within a 15 minute treatment, my dad was suffering from angina and after one 4 day treatment not only had the symptoms vanished but when the doctors went to check his heart from inside they could not find anything anymore.

A little girl with Leukemia came for one 4 day treatment and tests a month after showed they were free of it… there are countless results, I'm not sure I can class them as Level I,II or beyond but the work ethic most certainly changes, its not just, "wow this is powerful, look what happens", but more a calling and responsibility, like it changed patients and family's life it also changed mine!

Having experienced both 1-on-1 treatments and the group, I now suggest to all the clients calling up for treatments to join the group, so they can experience the sheer power of it! In LA a woman suffering from Parkinson's came with a debilitating pain in her heal, it cleared by the time it was her turn to receive her first treatment. When you see a man come in in a wheelchair and push the chair out after his treatment it moves people, it gives them hope and see the light, if it can happen for him they will believe it can happen to themselves. In a group there is no need to talk about results or how great the method is, the proof is in front of all of us, we will see it happen!

The method is structured in such a clear and simple way that therapists are able to work together even if they don't speak the same language, nothing matters but the result and the clinics have proven that over and over for the past 10 years.

The seminars are structured in the same clear and simple way! How else could someone go away after 20 hours of training, learning about techniques and protocols and treat someone with angina, a stroke, MS or cancer and have a great result!

This method will demand you leave the ego behind and allow the energy to do it's work, it holds the blueprint of health, hence knows exactly what's needed! Follow the simplest of simple instructions and you will have success! Level I students go away and are amazed that they can have the results they have, what more do we need to say, it all speaks for itself!

Taking the seminars has changed my life and it's still changing but in a good way, the trust I developed in the method and in my teacher was instantaneous. It happened the moment I watched the healing documentary film 'Think About It', and I have never looked back. So what if I had paid a lot of money for other courses, it helped me to find this method of Bioenergy Healing. All I can say is thank you for that!

Students at the seminar also experience healing...

A wonderful course that has left me with a great feeling of well being, confidence and looking forward to building a successful practice. While on the course the following little things healed:

A gum infection disappeared

A skin complaint on my thumb healed and returned to normal (it had been that way for at least 4 months)

A cut on my cheek which continuously got infected and had failed to heal since August has healed completely

Finally I've been trying to eliminate Athletes foot for the past 2 years and that has now completely gone also.

Why I love practicing the method .... feeling like Superman ...

Two of the main laws of Nature are: "The law Of Giving", and " The Law of Cause and Effect".

To me, giving someone Bioenergy Treatments and help them heal from some illness is the most precious form of giving.

The first treatment I gave to my wife when I came back from Level 1 Seminar and to my big surprise ... IT WORKED. She had sore feet and after one treatment, the pain disappeared. Was I ever happy and a little bit surprised, but it gave me lots of confidence. My wife still didn't believe I had much to do with it, but she was happy that her feet did not hurt any more. (She became a "believer", after she attended with me the Level 2 in Seattle.)

After that, I helped a few relatives and friends with allergies, back pain, migraine, emotional issues, sciatica and vertigo and everyone I treated was healed.

The most amazing experiences were when I helped an 8-year-old boy and 23 year old girl from Croatia, get rid of their allergies. The Boy was taking allergies pills for 6 years and girl for 20 years, and I helped them get rid of them in 8 treatments. Wow, was I exited.... Can you believe it, I was in California and they were in Croatia? I felt like a Superman.

Also, when I was on vacation in Croatia, I met a nice lady from Bosnia that had a stroke 3 years ago. She could not pronounce any words properly, she could not walk because her right leg was bent and she could not open her right fist.

Well, after 4 in person therapies and 20 long distance therapies, she can pronounce many words properly, and she can walk by herself. Her fist opened completely after first therapy and closed again, but not completely like before. Her husband told me that she is so exited about the treatments and results that she can hardly wait for her treatment and after that she goes for a walk for hrs.. She has never been late one minute for her treatment. Doing her treatments gives me lots of positive energy and motivation.

As far as "The law of Cause and Effect/Action and Reaction" that I mentioned at the beginning, her husband told me that I can stay in their hotel on Adriatic Sea whenever I want and as long as I want. Who says that laws of nature don't work?

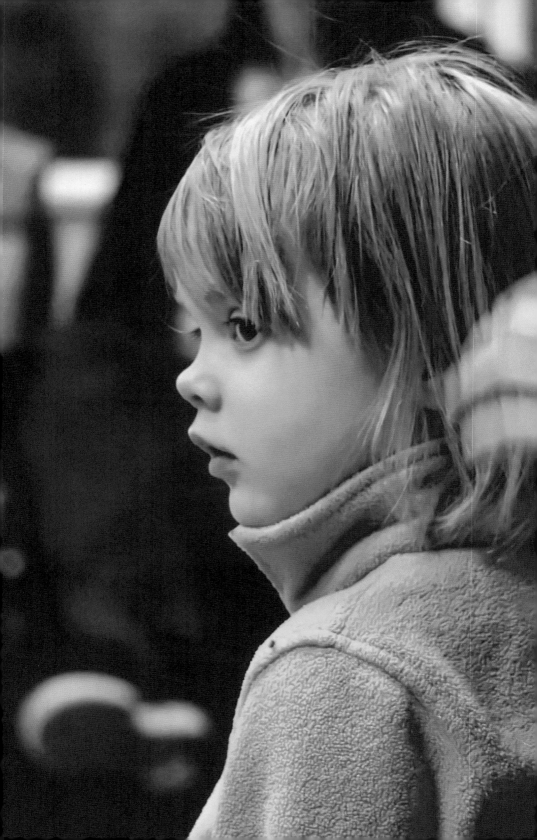

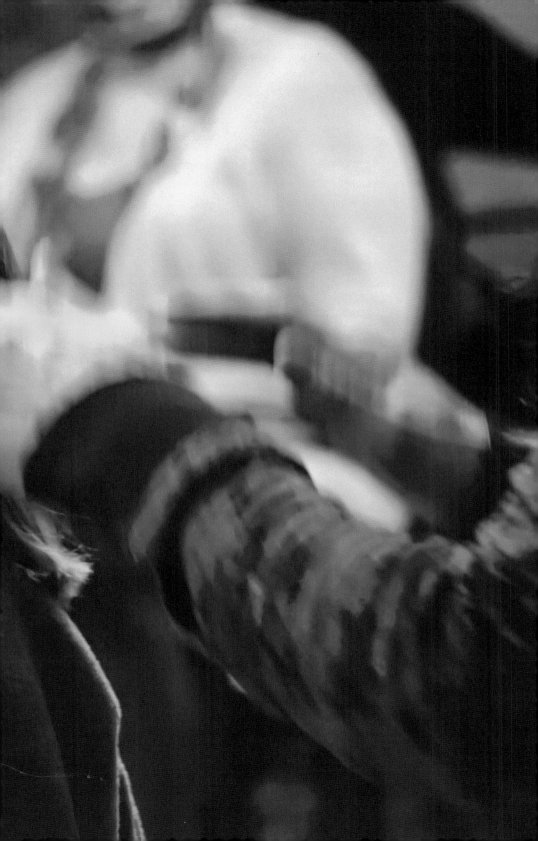

Why I love practicing the method (short blogs)

"I feel part of something I can't explain with words.

....

"Energy is moving and changing my body, opening my mind and touching my spirit. It's linking me back with something wonderful and unfathomable. I am instantly connected and whole. That feeling is spilling into other areas of my life and helping me look at everything with different eyes."

....

"Going to the beach" is where I go. We have a place in Naples, FL that we stay at for 10 days at a time, from Guelph, Ontario, about 5 times per winter. So when I'm working with a client, that's where I go. I fly fish, I walk the beach, I visit the pier, I go to our favourite birding spots, etc. So I have similar feelings in both situations: happy, excited, engaged with life.When I'm being treated I choose to go to the beach rather than anything else. Wonderbar."

....

"Why not, it is LOVE and LIFE itself! When you can give a gift like this, how can you feel anything but great about what your doing!

This is a great opportunity for people to really help others. Because of this it seems to attract people that think the same way as you do. We have been given a beautiful gift. One that needs to be shared.

Thank you so much for the knowledge and guidance Zoran and Stephanie!"

....

"Healing Bioenergy is a way of showing gratitude to the world around you. Caring for others is a huge step the gifts that we can give each other. The more you do it, the more gratitude you feel for the opportunity to share this healing technique and to be able to help so many at once. There are not too many things in life that give you such a big return for your kindness, and this is one of them."

....

"For me I feel really peaceful, happy and in a Zen state of mind. I'm present for the person I´m working on but also in a mindless state at the same time, I guess you could call it selective awareness... :)

Sometimes I feel the energy flowing in me and sometimes my hands feel hot and tingly especially when doing long distance.

I haven´t had any therapy done on me so I can´t comment on that aspect, but I look forward to that experience !

Also I still feel a moment or two every session I do of gratitude to be on this path, and for both Zoran and yourself for making the teachings available outside of Europe."

....

"When I'm practising Bioenergy Therapy on a patient, it feels like time stands still. Everything seems to slow down and I always get a wonderful, profound feeling of stillness, love & kindness around me. It feels like there is a very powerful healing & loving presence surrounding the patient and I. Best of all, the patient's pain levels drop dramatically after 1 session in 90% of Treatments! A truly amazing therapy!"

....

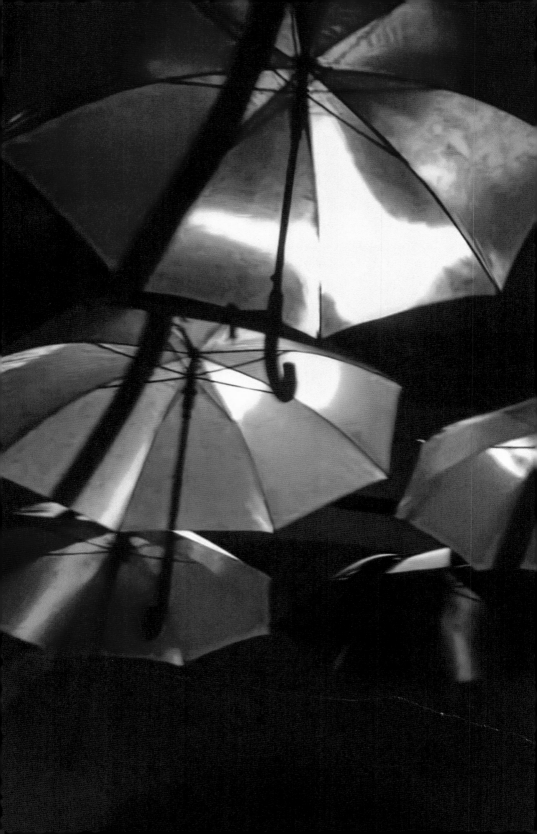

benefits of the group

Therapy with PUREBIOENERGY™ can be practiced in person, one on one, non-locally, at a distance and in a group. Its true potential often resonates best with people when performed in a group.

PUREBIOENERGY™ experienced in a group provides yet another dimension to the healing process, magnifying it through group dynamics.

The "group energy" changes over the course of the four days and a real sense of community is created. As the days progress people really open up and are interacting with each other. They recognize all of the changes that happen with each other, increasing the effect of the event.

Four days in a row allows the physical body to "catch up" with the energy body and a repetition of the same process magnifies the abilities to achieve the body's self-healing potential.

Science proved that, besides strenghtening the belief system, witnessing directly boosts the immune system, which is the only way to restore the original well-being.

Relationship and interaction between practitioners also adds to the success of the healing event. The effect of experienced bioenergists working together, within the group, is many times greater than the sum of its parts and the benefits of the method become intensified.

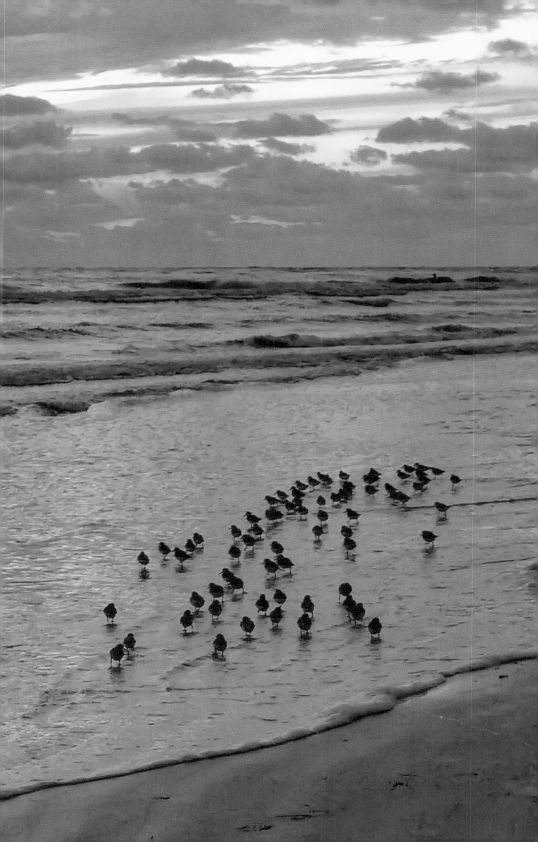

Group

Client feedback from London clinic

"Thank you for the wonderful experience we had, it was so good to see all the people in good health and smiling from the day 2... my friends and I have gained full health. No more kidney pain and bladder problems for one of my friends, the hospital visits are a thing of the past now. The other friend got his swollen knee back to normal just after the first treatment and his hearing improved to everybody's delight. The other friend got her lupus and arthritis and cysts gone.... My varicose veins are gone and cyst on the back of my head gone, sinus inflammation gone.... Thank you million times Sonja, there are no words to describe how grateful we are and see you soon for another PureBioenergy healing"

Glimpse of a group clinic

ASTHMA - 2 children aged 4 and 6 are free of asthma symptoms after 2 treatments. They are sleeping through the night and in no need of any medication or inhalers!

Their mum suffering from ANKYLOSING SPONDYLITIS is free of pain after many years of constant pain and agony, her BLOOD PRESSURE is also back to normal and she was telling us yesterday that for the first time in ages she was running after the kids not even realising until they told her that she is!!! Looking at her walking in even her depression had gone, all smiles and happiness!

Everyone is loving the children in the group, they accept treatments without judgment and it shows in their incredibly fast results! An inspiration needless to say!

All patients suffering from ARTHRITIS and RHEUMATOID ARTHRITIS are free of pain, most of them after their first ever treatment!

ALLERGIES and SINUS PROBLEMS gone!

A young woman suffering from MULTIPLE SCLEROSIS is free of symptoms, walking without pain, not ridged anymore rather fluid movements and EVERYbody in the group realises. The stiffness in her fingers has lifted and strength has come back!

RAYNAUD'S DISEASE CLEARING, no more itchy toes during the night, not affected by temperature changes anymore, circulations overall improved, patient came in wearing flip flops yesterday with a big smile on her face

SPINAL INJURY from a tumor operation left a patient in agony and not being able to walk properly, that cleared within 2 days, it turned his life around he says. His Tennis Elbow is almost 100% better!

August London clinic results

A woman with (for her) embarrassingly red feet and hands (doctors could not diagnose what it was), chronic fatigue, pain in elbows and lower back had a bit of a healing crisis during the first treatment, saying she had enough or her body had enough... she understood what I said about the 4 days being a process and the body resisting change sometimes and I am sure she is glad she stayed as EVERY-thing shifted almost all in the first session! We could literally see the colour in her hands disappearing. On day 4 she didn't wear socks and even had her nails painted. She was so happy as she remembered that she didn't go back to Yoga because the teacher made her take her socks off and she was so embarrassed about her red toes.

She even brought in her dog on Day 3, who had some traumatic experience at a dog kennel when they last went on holiday, the dog wouldn't leave her sight. After just a short treatment he refused to leave the clinic... she even left the venue so the dog didn't see her anymore and that didn't make a difference either. Apparently that was the ultimate test, the lady said. The dog laid down and feet up in the air for more intake of BioEnergy. You can imagine EVERYbody loved that! On Day 4 the dog was hiding from his owner after the treatment, wanted to stay again ;-))))

Another amazing case of Arthritis in literally ALL joints reduced by over half after the first treatment, the lady has never taken pain-killers or any other medication prescribed by doctors, she managed pain through meditating which took up a lot of her time as you can imagine. By Day 2 she could hardly believe how much time she had on her hands because she didn't have to manage the pain. What was extraordinary in her case was that she couldn't stretch her legs as her knees were in so much pain, but on Day 2 she stretched them AND couldn't believe her eyes. No Pain at all either.

A lady with Emphysema wouldn't be able to walk 5 meters without the use of Oxygen and after the 1st treatment she walked 200m to the car, part of it uphill and NO problem at all ;-) Her second issue was a bright light in the corner of her eye and that cleared up within minutes.

The lady with Liver Cancer and tumors on Lungs and ribcage will beat her cancer with the help of bioenergy, no more chemo, she had enough of the side effects. Her IBS went away in the 4 days, from after her first treatment she had colour in her face and said this is exactly what she was praying for and she is confident that she will be healthy, then she went home and signed up for all the clinics to the end of this year ;-)

"Healing so subtle yet so drastic" - Client feedback

From Maine clinic

"It has been two full weeks since my Bio Energy Healing in Water-ville. I am having difficulty articulating what happened to me, but I have had healing on many levels of consciousness. I will start by saying if you can't comprehend this form of healing it probably isn't for you....I am no longer suffering panic/anxiety. I am no longer living in a heightened state of anxiety/fear over everything. I have an awareness about the escalating thought patterns that escalate my emotions to panic, AND I now have an ability to see in my mind an alternative to panic! This healing is changing my chronic pain problem on a daily basis, and it goes without saying that someone who has been living with fear, panic, anxiety, PTSD etc. behaves dif-ferently, makes better choices when they are not caught in that state of mind!!!! Don't misunderstand or misinterpret me here, I am still reaching 58 in a few days so my body has not returned to 20 any-thing, but I feel better and am using less pain meds and see a better future for myself with my health....

If you are thinking to yourself about your life, your health, your body mechanics, your psychic state of mind, etc. that " there must be another way"! There is, it is PUREBIOENERGY Healing.

This healing is so subtle, yet so drastic, it is very difficult to explain. I have been stuck/ experiencing a vicious cycle of pain, panic, anxiety for so long that "I" "Me" has been lost in all of that for such a long time that I keep thinking and feeling like "I am back!" I have the ability to not panic. This is a miracle for me. Life transforming for certain. The future looks very bright!"

Group insight from the L.A. healing event

"On the other side of the room, Zoran works on a young woman whose hands are shaking uncontrollably. Like attracted by a magnet, her body moves slowly towards Zoran's hands.

Unseen ties seem to lift her head, shoulders and chest and she steps into the open space following her stretched arms. Her hands are steady. No tremor. She bursts into tears, dancing and waving her hands in the air, for all of us to see.

In the following two days, moments like the one described above multiply. The energy in the room becomes nurturing and stable. People talk to each other, exchange impressions and compliment each other's signs of improvement. The lack of privacy of the treatment space becomes a huge benefit. Emotionally, we participate to each other's healing. We become an inseparable part of this energy field that supports and unites us.

At the end of the third or forth session, D., a woman in her mid fifties who came from Sacramento, starts dancing. It was one of her dreams, after she was diagnosed with Parkinson's. She moves gently through the space, enjoying her flexibility and harmony.

It was only a day or two ago when she told me how embarrassed she felt for being ill. There is no discomfort in her dance now. Something magical has been awakened in her. Maybe self-confidence. Maybe hope. She seems ready to become her own healer.

Later on, I watch K. who only two days ago was totally immobilized in her wheelchair like in a cage. The caretaker who accompanied her was lifting her legs, one by one, to move them from one uncomfortable position to another. And here she is now, after the fifth or sixth session, smiling and rubbing her palms together as she saw the healers doing. Her face is relaxed and bright. Helped by her caretaker and one of the healers she lifts her body out of the wheelchair stretching herself upwards. She takes few timid steps into the unknown of health. We all applaud frantically."

Group event in Sarasota

She came in walking with a cane and after treatment she got up and said, "Mr. Pain is gone!"

The most impressive moment for me was when a certain gentleman came in in a wheelchair and, I think it was the very next day, he walked across the room without any assistance. That was wonderful for me to see.

I don't know her name but Zoran was working with her and he just pulled her back towards him and then leaned her forward and I just never saw anything like that. It was almost like hypnosis but I know it wasn't hypnosis. She was just very sensitive of his energies. It was the wildest thing I ever saw.

It has just been an unique experience, the team is really good, I am amazed about the amount of time, effort and energy that everybody is just putting in, It's just unbelievable, a lot of energy, a lot of work.

Another benefit, the one for my soul was seeing transformations that happened to people.

I loved the group because to see people when they first walk in the door and then to see what happens to them day by day, it's profound. It's a gift to be able to participate in this.

I started crying when Jean Harry started walking. I've known him for a long time. I pushed that man in a wheelchair since April. He couldn't get out of his chair. It was pretty amazing. Yes, that was the outstanding moment.

Everybody should know about this. Seriously, there has to be a way to let people know about this. If people knew there would be lines out the door. Who wouldn't want this?

Honestly, I was thinking that I would come to this event just one day, I didn't know what to expect, I didn't realize it was four days and I wish I could have maybe gone longer but I felt it was important enough to come back the second time just because of changes that I felt from one treatment. It is encouraging how I felt yesterday and today.

Just the kinda vibe, you know, there is a lot of people injured, and seeing how happy everyone was, the feeling that you got from being around for just the short time was definitely impressive. It is nice that there are people around willing to help and that really impressed me the most.

When my daughter moved down here in November she was wheelchair bound, years without being able to work, she's been bedridden for long periods of time, she has done all kinds of things and today I saw something unique, not only did I see her jump today but the whole day she was in high heels. OK, this is new, she is walking in heels. This is cool. The first day after the session with Zoran she told me that the deep seeded ache in all of her joints was gone. It creeped back a little bit on a second day, eased again on a third day and today she is in high heels. She's glowing. What are you doing?

I stopped taking MSM, which kept me mobile, and I haven't seen a regression from stopping taking it. I feel terrific.

There has been a lot of release and also there has been a lot of breakthroughs and I know that it is going to continue to do its work and I feel it working when I go home. It is really a wonderful process.

Being able to do this continuously would be a great thing.

People doing the energy work were wonderful and caring.

By coming here I learned that giving is a wonderful thing and we should be doing more of that.

From Bioenergy Life Center healing event in London

We had such an incredible healing event in London; Child's Diabetes is on its way out. Reading in the morning of Day 1 was 11 and on Day 3 it was at 6.

30 yrs. of excruciating Arthritis pain (using 8 tablets of pain

medication to numb the pain) literally went within the first treatment.

Side effects of Radio Therapy cleared up on Day 1, another patient's side effects of Chemo (nausea, headaches, skin flaking off, itching, digestion not working, tiredness...) went away by Day 2, and she was so much happier and more energetic, looking forward to the rest of her life!

Injury pains that never cleared up even after OP, leaving this woman in constant pain, with swollen legs and ankles. The pain was gone after 3 minutes of working on the area of neuropathy in her leg. The swelling was gone completely by Day 3 and on Day 4 she came in looking radiant, happy and thanking us for changing her life and that of her family. She wants to take the training course in February to help her family with whatever ailments they have.

Another cancer patient reported that the lymph nodes that were hurting and swollen are not hurting anymore. The lump in her breast is minimal. Sleeping better, felling better in herself and on top of it her back pain she never mentioned until the last day has gone, too!

Blood pressure is back to normal after 2 Days of treatments. The list goes on!

A child, born with a heart condition, won't need the second open-heart surgery; doctors can't quite believe it but is a fact, as the tests show clear improvement!

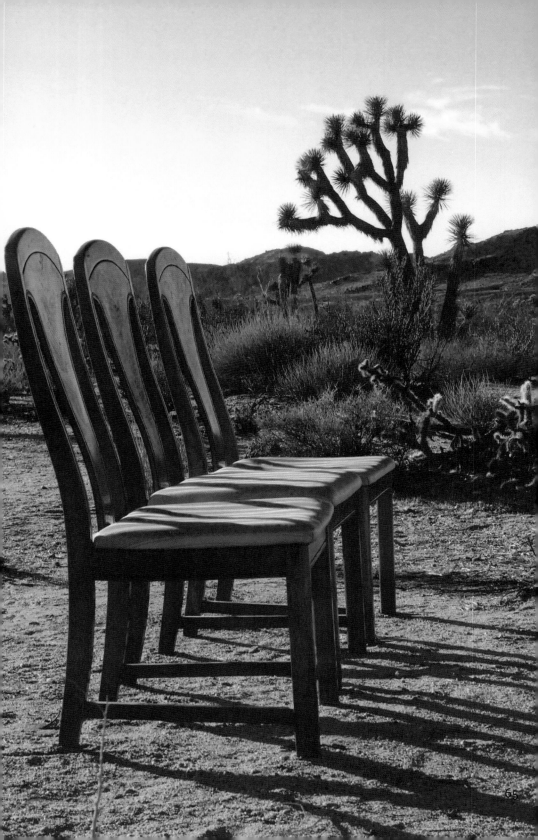

you can do it anywhere

How about the beach? Or a parking lot, for that matter?

Bioenergy, since it is a self-contained bundle of information, can be, and it is, used anywhere.

Unless you are a professional healer you don't need a special designated space. There is no need for a temple, hospital, office, retreat, yoga mat or massage table. If you know how to channel this energy, it will go through your hands no matter where you are.

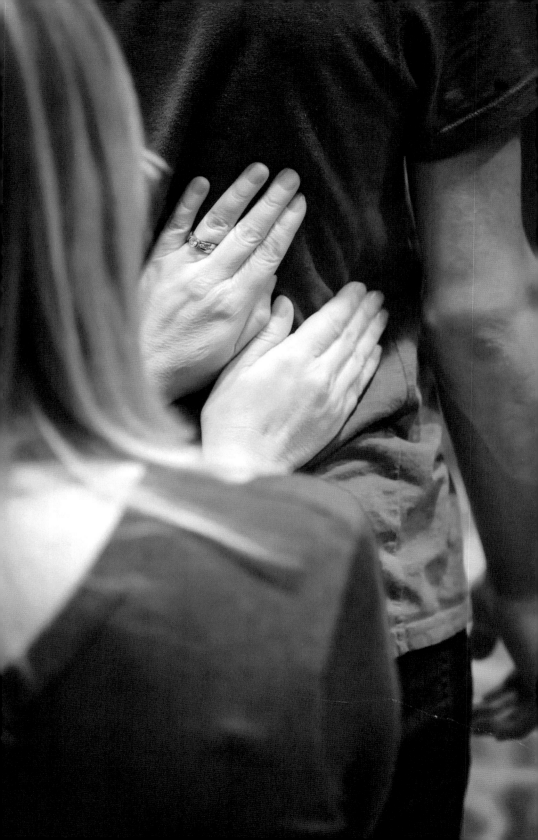

Some Results - by Condition

Allergies

Allergy, Sweden — 17 yr old

I have now done 2 healing sessions on the 17 year old girl with the egg and soya allergy. The first time she reacted very strongly emotionally and cried every time when I did the healing, but on the 4th day she looked so clear and happy. We have now just finished the second session and she says "her stomach is better, she really likes the healing and just to test the airborne egg-allergy, she has walked outside restaurants and bakeries where she normally reacts with runny nose and eyes, and now has no reaction at all. Stomach is much better and today she told me that a teacher came running after her and was wondering - what is happening? The teacher has noticed something changing in her and she looks much more healthy.

Second time she didn't react that emotionally as first time, just a little cold but now she was preparing for hockey.

In the end she asked me if I thought she will be able to learn this healing some day. Of course she will :)

Sinus allergy symptoms gone

Today is 11th day since our last session Thursday and here is how I feel now and felt during this period. Friday I felt little bit better than usual. Next day I was 'worse', my nose was running like crazy but it wasn't stuffed/clogged as much as it used to be. Sunday felt OK. I 'survived' whole day by spraying the nose only twice in almost 24hr period. Monday morning after I woke up my nose was stuffed a bit but nothing I could not stand like it used to be. I went to the gym, did my exercise, all other stuff, went to work, basically the day was passing by and I felt good. Finally, the day was over. I went to bed around midnight with my nose clear. I was surprised and happy that whole day passed and I did not need to use stupid nose spray. Now it gets really interesting :)...... my nose has been clear ever since and today is 7th day since I have no more allergy symptoms. Occasional sneezing happens through the day but those few sneezes through the whole day I would consider normal for any person even without the allergy. I feel really good and beyond happy! THANK YOU!!! I hope this will last...

Zoran, thank you very much again for all your help and assistance! I feel like a healthy person again. I had no doubts about your work even before we started but I do have to admit that I was getting worried I might not be lucky enough to react to the therapy for whatever reason. I never thought in my life that I will be so happy saying I WAS WRONG :)

Arthritis/Joints/Spine

Chronic Arthritis gone and still gone after 2 years

Just got a letter from a client that I treated 2 years ago for chronic arthritis. She had very painful right knee and hip for more than 15 years, and it was getting worse. The pain went down, and disappeared by the 4th day of therapy, and she could walk fine. After 2 weeks she felt pain creeping back, and we did another 4 days.

Today, she writes: "Well, You really fixed my knee, and hip!

I didn't have any problems since our treatments.

I was kinda waiting for the pain and stiffness to come back, but they didn't!"

Arthritis in feet, neck, lower back

"For years I have been suffering with severe arthritis on my feet, neck and lower back. I have been on pain medication for the past 9 years. I have seen several specialists: Foot specialist, orthopedic and rheumatologist and they all told me that there was not much help other than pain medication. I went to a Bioenergy Therapist as a last resort and, after four day healing session, I am happy to say that I am off the pain medication. My energy level has grown greatly and I feel I can walk again. Thank you! You have made my life so much better! Sincerely, E."

Bursitis

"I treated a man with bursitis and he had the x rays done afterwards and even the bone spurs were gone so he had to make up a story for the doctors who were kind of shocked."

Gnarled Hands

Have a client that has hands like gnarled tree roots, all twisted, inflamed, red and very, very painful.

She was an accomplished pianist and teacher but reduced to limited teaching only.

After 2 treatments (8 x sessions) she is happily back to teaching and is able to play Chopin's Ballade in G minor, apparently one of the most difficult pieces to play. She is over the moon.

Neck pain and rosacea….

"I feel so blessed to have you in my life! You gave me such a gift of healing from the constant pain I have been suffering that ran from the right side of my neck, through my right shoulder and down my arm. After each healing session I always noticed more and more relief until all of a sudden I was unconsciously using the vacuum and it didn't hurt! Then It hit me like WOW! The pain is totally gone! I couldn't wait to tell you. I am so excited and overwhelmed with gratefulness! And that's not the only blessed thing that happened, as my Rosacea cleared up as well!

I am spreading my joy around about what you have done for me as I have tried other modalities that kind of worked, but what you have learned and are practicing is truly a gift of absolute healing."

Off pain medicine – after 3 years

"Three months ago, I started taking a new anti-inflammatory drug to alleviate the pain and stiffness in my joints – primarily in my hands, wrists and hips – and found that within a week there was a significant decrease in pain… However I began to experience some ugly side effects, one serious enough to bring me to the ER. Against my doctor's advice, I stopped taking the medication. A week later, I was experiencing all the same aches and pains all over again. I then decided to attend a Bioenergy Therapy group. By the third day, I noticed that I was feeling much better and the pain had shifted from a sharp acute pain that would linger for hours to more like rapid spams. It has been four days since I completed the Group Healing Treatment; I have not had any significant pain or discomfort in my joints and I am feeling more energetic! This is especially important to me because this is the first time in 3 years that I am completely off of any medication and I feel fine. I feel a great sense of relief and peacefulness inside and have a better understanding of the emotional pain that still haunts my soul from time to time. I feel a good 'vibe' all around."

Osteoporosis / Bone Density and multiple results

Daughter helps Mom in many ways - from relieving Rheumatoid Arthritis to improving bone density and more

Her daughter says, "It's like her immune system is finding more and more ways to use the energy now that so many of the old painful issues have cleared up."

Here is their story:

A mother with borderline bone density issues just found out her most recent bone scan shows "significant improvement" over the last one! She had done nothing to address this issue, but has been having periodic rounds of Purebioenergy healing over the past 9 months from her daughter. They started by focusing on her Rheumatoid Arthritis, but expanded out to cover some of her additional issues over time...This feels special for the mother because most of her early rounds were to treat flaring arthritis, bursitis, shingles, joints so deformed they would split the skin if she bent them too much, decades of insomnia, decades of anxiety, overwhelming seasonal allergies, sciatica, back pain, painful tailbone, etc....Almost all of those issues are now gone, so the daughter started focusing on the "smaller" problems that are part of her overall health picture like high blood pressure, heel spurs, weak wrists, weak knees, etc. "We are still working on some deformed joints and RA issues at the same time, but now she is seeing more and more of these "side benefit" improvements that were not directly related to what she asked to have treated (bone density)".

Scoliosis results with x-rays

I just wanted to say thank you so much for the treatment! I went to the healing session in Seattle in April 3-6 for scoliosis and just went in for an x-ray. The curve in the lower part of my back reduced from 31 to 24 degrees and my spine has started to rotate back into the correct position! The chiropractor I go to said that such improvements are usually seen only after 6 months.

Thank you,

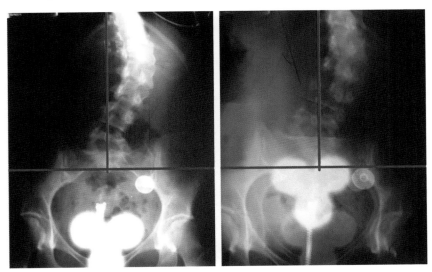

Curve reduced from 31 to 24 degrees

Back pain - 100% success rate

Since I have been using this method of bioenergy therapy for back pain, I have had a 100% success rate, and this covers a dozen cases of various, more or less chronic conditions: middle back pain, lower back (lumbago), upper back pain.

Some people can't help smiling at beginning of a session. (One patient asked "Are you chasing flies?") But 15 or 20 minutes later, to their own astonishment, it's 100% gone.

New Client with Sciatica

So the other day I had a 61 years old woman come to me because she had bad lower back pain from Sciatica. This woman knew absolutely nothing about BioEnergy, but she was willing to give it a try since the doctors could not help her manage the pain. She gave the first day a try and let's just say that she walked out speechless, with a big smile on her face and completely pain free!

The very next day I had received a phone call from her telling me that that evening was the first time in years she was able to go to the store and not have to use a motorized scooter or a shopping cart for support! So glad to see that BioEnergy is helping her out :)

Degenerative Disc Disease

For several years I had been struggling with what was diagnosed by doctors as degenerative disc disease. Then a few years ago I had fallen down the stairs in a weird split, which twisted my pelvis, herniated 2 discs in my lower back and landed on my left elbow - which over time grew stiff and finally went up and created a frozen shoulder. The doctor said they could surgically go into my shoulder and cut the muscles to release it. The doctor also told me I would probably be in pain the rest of my life, with my pelvis and lower back, and gave me life long subscriptions to acupuncture, chiropractor, and pain meds to manage the pain.

Previously, I was in the military and dealt with a variety of major imbalances in my body and never seemed to recover. For instance I didn't have a period for 2 years, then I had one for 6 months straight. Essentially I was out of balance and constantly felt like an emotional mess.

I tried a number of things over the years, however nothing really worked long term. I always just knew there had to be something that could help reverse these things I was living with, I couldn't accept just learning to live with it. I stumbled on Bioenergy Therapy and signed up for the course and a PureBioenergy healing treatment with Zoran Hochstatter.

After one session I noticed some improvements such as sleeping a full 9 solid hours with out waking up in pain or tossing and turning and most of the pain was relieved (I had not had a solid night of sleep in two years prior to the first session). After session two, 75% of my pain was gone. By day three in early a.m.- I had a massive emotional release, which was a combination of cry and hysterical laughing. By the end of day three I had no pain in my body at all what so ever. The important thing to note in this story is not just that I had no pain, but that for the first time in years my back actually felt STRONG, balanced and stable. I could just walk normal and felt confident that I could just walk and not worry about a mis-step throwing my back out. By session four - I felt a sense of peace that I hadn't felt in such a long time I had forgotten what it was to be internally calm, I mean really at peace and clear headed. It felt like I had a total reset emotionally and physically and that I was in perfect balance.

As time passed and I continued to do this PureBioenergy Therapy work with my own clients, I saw many internal and external things in my life that were once in conflict coming to resolution. Prior to doing this work, I was unable to even recognize that there were any conflicts. My thought patterns changed and my whole out look on life completely changed. Today, I'm at peace on the inside of myself, regardless of what's happening around me. I'm calmer and more emotionally capable of observing and handling difficult situations without becoming upset or totally engrossed in the drama of the situation. I'm able to look at a situation happening and step into a more observatory role in the situation with out getting caught up in it. I still have emotions of course, but I don't stress about small stuff, In fact I can't think of much I stress about at all anymore. I'm more honest with myself about my own thoughts and behaviors, and I feel I'm more honest with others. People that haven't seen me in a while tell me that my eyes look clearer, and I seem different, I look younger, I seem calmer and less erratic emotionally.

Autoimmune

Lupus Healing Story

The wife of a friend of mine was diagnosed with Lupus. The medications she was given were not easing her pain, nor did the diet and dietary supplements recommended by her nutritionist. Her husband convinced her to try Bioenergy Therapy.

Two weeks after following the protocol for Lupus for 4 consecutive

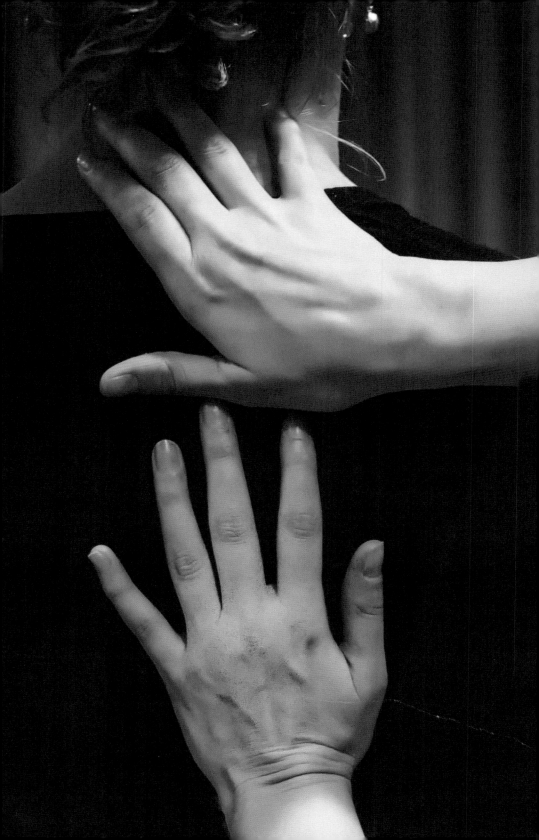

days, she went to her doctor for some lab work. She said the doctor came into the exam room with her previous lab results in one hand, and the results from that day's lab work in the other. He looked back and forth from one hand to the other and exclaimed, "These dates are backwards!"

After comparing the current lab results with the previous results for a bit longer, he placed both papers on the counter, looked at my friend and announced, "You don't have Lupus, anymore." Then he simply walked out of the room.

Blood

Blood disease report

A client with a blood disease called ITP (low thrombocytes) for five years now has had constant problems with bleeding in all forms since that, mostly nose bleeds. Doctors took the spleen away and for a while he stopped bleeding. Last Christmas it was so bad that the doctors wanted to put him on cortisone and eventually blood transfusion at the hospital (blood platelets was 20). He refused and tried other methods with natural medicines and nutrition. He made some small progress but the great response is now after 4 sessions of Bioenergy healing during a 5 months period.

The last 3 months he has only had 2 nose bleeds.

Yesterday he had some tests done at the hospital and the blood platelets are now 85, best ever since many years, and he is happy!!

Cholesterol level down

Just wanted to share with everyone about a treatment I gave to a patient who had a cholesterol level of 7.9 and I did the four day treatment working on her liver and she just called me as she went for a test the day after her fourth treatment and her level is now 5.1!!!!!! Her doctor wanted to prescribe statins and still can't believe it and wants her to have another test.

Cancer

Breast cancer results

I have done one breast cancer patient who also had cysts in the same breast and even though the pain was gone after the first round of 4 she wanted to do another round. We did that and she had a thermogram done which showed NO tumours or cysts or hot spots. This was a phenomenal experience of the Bioenergy Therapy which was able to be confirmed by a Naturopath on many different levels by a machine she had.

A patient was referred to me for a tumour as well as heart "squeezing" episode along with extreme exhaustion with low drop of blood pressure which sent her to the hospital where they could not give her an answer. I found the answer through muscle testing her and did Bioenergy for her. On the 2nd day she said she felt invincible already and could not believe how she was feeling. She said every day she woke up she felt as if someone was laying on her body and it was all she could do to drag herself out of bed. When she had the test on the device after the two rounds of Bioenergy therapy her cancer markers were 20 something as opposed to the 222 before the treatment. Her naturopath asked her what had she been doing to get the numbers down so low in such a short time. [Both sessions were done close together] ... Such beautiful results able to be verified--oh yeah--also hot spots showed on thermogram of muscles that were injured in arm and shoulder blade area that we added bioenergy and there was nothing there after the therapy.

Another patient had long distance therapy for bad sores in both breasts and the doctors wanted to take her breasts off. We did 2 rounds of Bioenergy and they did not have to remove the breasts!

Cancer Healing Story

In 2012 , I trained with Zoran and completed my seminar 1 & 2 and was practicing for 18 months having amazing results. Then in December 2013, I went to the doctor with a tummy upset , which much to my horror, was initially diagnosed as Grade 3 metastatic ovarian cancer. I had gone from fit and healthy with no symptoms to dying over night!!!! The first person I contacted was Zoran . He started remote healing on 5th January 2014 and after major debulking surgery on 15th January he did a second session. By day 2 the terrible swelling in my abdomen caused by the surgery had gone, my energy levels were up and my pain went completely AND never came back!!!

He continued to treat me until April and by June I was according to my doctor in full remission. I got better and better. Sadly in September it came back and after further tests it became clear that I had been misdiagnosed. I actually had stage 4 stomach cancer which had spread into my abdomen. Again I contacted Zoran and he has supported me with healing through my treatment.

If it wasn't for his help and support I wouldn't be here to tell this story. My doctors are amazed that the disease has improved and I am stable. I can't thank Zoran enough he is amazing and continuing to support me on my journey to complete health. My heart felt thank you for everything !!!

Disappearance of the ovarian tumor

"I am a professional violinist and I am 26 years old. I always travel a lot with my job and I am under a lot of stress due to my busy performance schedule. I can say that I have a very hectic life. About 5 months ago, following some routine medical check-up, my doctor discovered that I have a malignant tumor on my left ovary. I was very desperate at that moment but I regained my control and decided to do long distance bioenergy therapy. I did an intensive series of treatments. In only 2 months and a half of bioenergy therapy, medical test and ultrasound proved the disappearance of the ovarian tumor. I'm left without words, thank you so much."

Doctors gave this guy no chance with lung cancer in final stages

PureBioenergy Therapy works in mysterious ways,… we worked on a man for a tumour found on his left lung, the hospital and doctors told his wife and family to prepare for the worst, left him more or less to his own devices, horrendous to watch, heart breaking and everything else!

We started treating him twice a day for 4 days after the he got sent home as they said they couldn't do anything anymore. After these initial 4 days I did 4-day treatments for a month, then they decided on starting chemo,.. soon after his kidneys failed and again apparently no help.. when we of course knew his body was too weak to take the chemo... but of course we couldn't take this decision away from him..

After the first bioenergy treatment on the kidneys, they worked again the next morning, doctors couldn't believe it, thought they made a mistake,... we continued the healing for him, he got better and better, even though they couldn't do the chemo,..

After 2 weeks they allowed him to go home,... he had ups and downs of course, as he was fed on a drip and almost no solid food,.. his intestines had to learn to work again, the whole digestive system had to start all over, he got weaker and weaker, so they took him back to hospital thinking the cancer had spread and is weakening him, but then the news... they did an ultrasound on his kidneys where he had metastases, couldn't find anything anymore,... the tumor on his lung is considerably smaller, then the doc couldn't believe what he saw and ordered a CT scan which confirmed all of the above... now this guy is a convert, completely changed person,.. his doctor asked him what he was doing, as whatever they do in the hospital couldn't have caused this positive changes. He told him, to which the doctor replied, come back in a month, we do another test and then you go to the papers with this, as the whole world should know.

The story is so much longer and more detailed but I tried to squeeze it into a nutshell, so you can see what is possible...

Positive results on Lymphoma

Woman in her seventies with a history of lymphoma, water in her lungs and fatigue. This past spring she had chemo. She hadn't been feeling better during the summer and her doctor told her she might need stronger chemo next time.

After a series of 3 group healing sessions this autumn she had an appointment with her doctor today to see if she would indeed need more chemo. She called after the visit to her doctor. Her blood samples were very good, the protein which was way too high - 20 before was now normal -7, the water in her lungs almost gone, also the swollen lymph nodes much better. She only needs to come back in 3 months for a check-up. Her energy has gone way up with every group healing she´s attended. Needless to say she was very happy!

Diabetes

Diabetes and Hypertension

A 75 year old man with a long history of diabetes type 2 was treated long distance. After only one session his blood sugar was perfectly normal ....and not only that. When he checked up his blood pressure he discovered that also his hypertension was gone... I feel blessed to be able to help people with this method - so simple to learn and practice, and with such amazing results!

Diabetes Type 1 results

"A client came to me with Type 1 Diabetes and its consequences. He had been diabetic for the last 20 years, having to regulate his blood sugar level with twice-daily insulin injections for the last 2 years. I used the diabetes protocol on him for 4 days...Over the 2 weeks following bioenergy therapy, his blood sugar level slowly stabilized, and leveled off at normal! He no longer needed his injections, but still monitored himself just to make sure."

Ears

Deaf boy treated by Mom - Bioenergy Life Center UK

"Parents weren't aware of their son being deaf on one ear until he was getting behind in school. They have no idea if he was born like that and the doctors missed it or if it developed later on. Fact is he was deaf on that ear,... when I treated him in the clinic he got much more relaxed, they already saw huge improvement in his concentration and school work and he didn't want to wear the hearing aid anymore, it bothered him and so they removed it. After his Mom did the Level 1 Training she was treating him on a regular basis and as the following message shows, commitment pays off in a big way. "The Bioenergy Therapy has changed our lives! My son is not suffering from Lactose Intolerance anymore. And now the seemingly impossible is happening! He is starting to hear sounds with his 'deaf' ear. Thank you for this incredibly fascinating Level 1 Seminar!!"

Long-term loss of hearing

I would like to share the story of my very first client. My neighbor, at 18 years of age was in the U.S. Army serving in Vietnam when some artillery exploded in his foxhole, causing deafness. Although he was told he could return home, he stayed there out of concern for his fellow soldiers, and thus incurred additional hearing loss.

He is now in his early sixties, and the deafness has exacerbated into vertigo, tinnitus, and painful bouts of earaches. When I happened to see him shortly before my Level One class, he stated that he could not even hear with his hearing aid. I told him I would return the following Monday, and that he was welcome to be my first "guinea pig" client!

He arrived at my door shortly after I returned from the airport, and I used the protocol for ears. Even with the first session, he described a whirlwind moving around inside his head. Within four days, he stated that he could hear as well as he did when he was a teenager, without his hearing aid. The other symptoms cleared as well.

In two weeks, he returned for sessions for his allergies, which had made him "miserable" for thirty years, and most likely contributed to his ear symptoms. His allergies were cleared as well after the four days by using the Allergy protocol. He returns every couple of months for 4-day "tune-ups" on his ears.

Thank you to Zoran and Stephanie from the bottom of my heart for spreading and teaching the PUREBIOENERGY healing! I am so blessed to have this be a part of my life.

Meniere's disease

I just finished the first 4 day treatment for a client with Meniere's. I had this client give me an assessment for, both, Left and Right ears separately because the Left one has always been much worse than the Right. This client has been suffering with this ailment for over 23 years.

Day One we had a (Left) 40% improvement and (Right) 60% improvement for the remainder of the evening. Upon waking the next morning some nausea was present and both ears were back to their usual state of annoyance.

Day Two we had a (Left) 50% improvement and (Right) 70% improvement, also, for the remainder of the evening. Next morning both ears were close to being back to their usual state of annoyance but a little better. Client noticed the ability to laugh with her spouse on night 2, which she never does because the sound of laughter bothers her ears too much. Laughter = Success in this case! :)

Day Three we had a (Left) 40% improvement and (Right) 70% improvement for the remainder of the evening. Client tried to drive (which is usually difficult because of dizziness and the sound/movement of the other vehicles) & said she was able to go a short distance with minimal difficulty. Again, she was able to laugh and joke with her spouse! :)

Day Four we had a (Left) 60% improvement and (Right) 90% improvement. Client responded with this "I don't ever use the word 'Relaxed' or 'Calm' because it just isn't something that I feel in my ears or head.........not in over 23 years. But my Right ear went completely calm, completely relaxed, completely free! I don't know how to describe this feeling!" At this point, she almost has tears welling up from the feeling Biotherapy has given her.........What an AWESOME feeling for, both, her AND myself!

I LOVE having the ability to help others heal! What a truly incredible feeling!

Tone-deaf man truly healed — from BLC London

Treated a tone deaf client. He could lip read. I tested it during the first treatment, warming his lower back and he couldn't hear me asking him if the pain had gone down... on day 3 I asked quietly how his lower back felt and he answered.

This is what his wife wrote: "I'm feeling wonderful, truly healed. My husband is like a new man, not only has his knee complaint gone, but his hearing has improved ten fold, we are all truly inspired to spread the word of bio energy."

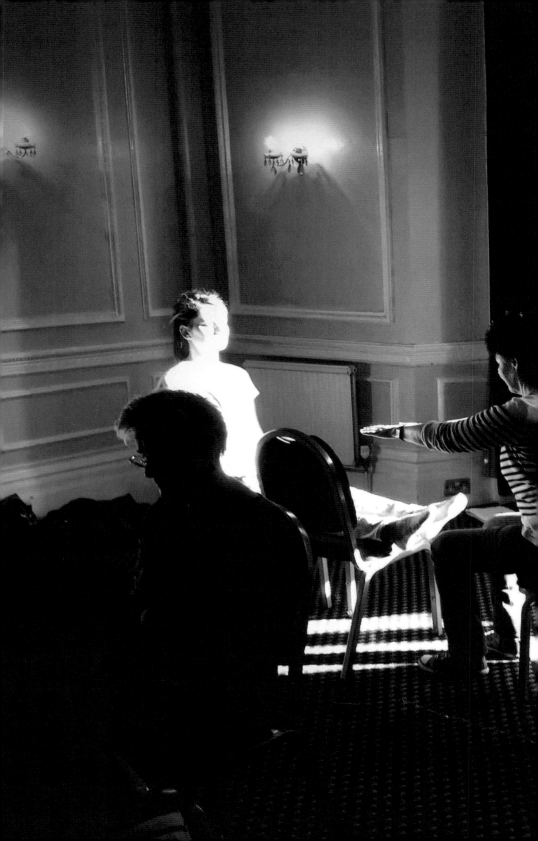

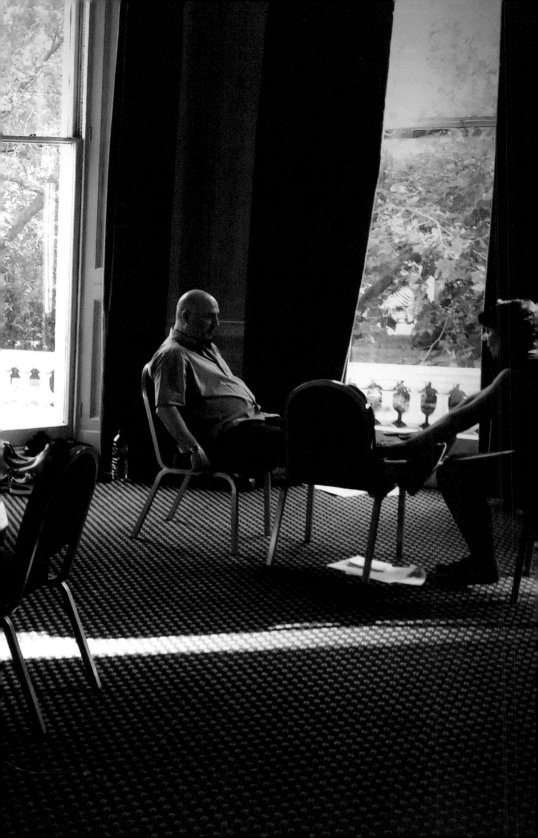

Eyes

Lazy eye and math

Since I had success with my daughter's lazy eye, I had someone else come to me for that. Hers was much worse. I mean, much!

Now get this.... due to her eye, she has always had real trouble with math as it seems that the numbers "move around" on her. Reading is hard, too. She has spent hours upon hours with a Math tutor. She still struggles to get 50% right on her tests.

After one 4 days treatment. her eye looked significantly better but got an email from her mother about 5 days later and it said, "Guess what??!!!! My daughter got an 88 on her math test!!!!!!!!!!!!!!!!!!!!!!!!!!!!" Yes she had that many exclamation points."

Glaucoma

"I started working with my mom (long distance) in March, and we did 4 days with 10 days rest (give or take a day) since then. Her first doctor gave her "bad news" and scheduled next visit for September... My sister took mom to another doctor after we had couple of treatments, and already her eye pressure was down to 15. After 3 more treatments Mom went for another checkup, and pressure is down to 11."

Macular degeneration

Someone I did eye therapy on six months back reported to me today the amazement of her eye specialist. She has macular degeneration in both eyes and had surgery and injections. At the follow up exam the doctor said her recovery was "remarkable". She said the doc said it was remarkable about three times. Her eyesight has since been stable.

Female Health

Free of hot flushes

All my clients suffering from severe hot flashes reported the following:

Dramatic decrease in hot flush frequency after 1 day of treatment.

Complete hot flash free after 3rd day, and uninterrupted sleep.

Most of them reported back to me every 10 days for more than 3 months. They are free of all symptoms they had before treatment.

Pap smear

"We don't always get 'results' feedback during the 4 day clinics we run. This week I ran into an attendee of one of the bioenergy clinics' previous 4 day events. That lady was keen to tell me that a week or so after the bioenergy clinic she attended, that she received medical results that indicated that for the first time in 10 years her cervical smear testing was normal. I asked did she think that the therapy helped, and she confirmed that she thought that was the case, that she was very surprised that the test were clear at all."

Thyroid and depression results

"In the 6 months since my level 2 training in San Diego I have been steadily working on patients with really amazing results. I seem to draw patients with similar issues. Many who suffer from depression, anxiety, panic attacks, insomnia, etc. - it is incredible how after one treatment it is gone! The other primary issue I seem to get is women with thyroid imbalances who are on medication. I've treated 5 women now for thyroid and every single one of them is off of their medication now, with perfectly normal functioning thyroids. I continue to be in awe of and humbled by this method, and I feel so much gratitude for your teachings and support."

Gastrointestinal

Constipation fixed - the awesomeness continues

I am very pleased with results so far. Feedback from the client on the second day was "I have got good news and really good news". The client has a tumour in his stomach and severe constipation. He hadn't had BM for five days and only a small one five days ago. His good news is he had BM this morning his really good news was that it was large, He is now really convinced that the method will help him with his cancer and asking if we can work on his Mercury poisoning next. The awesomeness continues.

Gallbladder patient

My toughest case responds. Since October of 2007, my 14 year old female patient has been vomiting several times a day. Not sick with nausea, just continuous vomiting. She was hospitalized and the CT/MRI finding was that the sphincter at the gall bladder was physically too small and positioned on an incline interfering with drainage.

The mother agreed with my advice that surgery was not the answer and wanted a second opinion at another Boston Hospital. She found a doctor who was willing to treat her conservatively. The vomiting continued. The doctors finally arrived at the conclusion that she did not respond to medical treatment and they were not positive on exactly what her problem was. They agreed to release her from care if the mother agreed to seek acupuncture care. I informed the mother that I was attending the Bio Energy healing seminar mainly to see if it would help her daughter. She was my first patient.

Three weeks after the first treatment the mother reports no vomiting for one whole week and counting. This is the most significant relief she has had since vomiting started in October. Vomiting was an everyday occurrence.

I share this case with you all because it demonstrates to me that the energy field was being addressed with this method of Bio Energy treatment that was not provided before. It showed me that it is something special and I personally am very grateful for the opportunity to have learned it and provide it to those in need.

Accident Recovery

Headaches after accident gone, no more meds

Around 6 weeks ago I treated the husband of a good friend of mine for severe, frequent and debilitating headaches due to a trapped nerve in the back of his neck after a bad fall 13 years ago. After a CT scan showed up nothing a year ago, he was prescribed anti-anxiety medication on top of the strong pain medication that he was taking on a daily basis anyway. Despite all this medication he still woke up a few times every night as he had to move his head and neck every 20 minutes as the pain would get worse.

On day 1, a few hours after the first session, he called to tell me he had an excruciating headache, worse than he had in a long time. I told him to take a pain killer and that he would be fine tomorrow as sometimes it gets worse before it gets better.

On day 2 he came and said the pain eased off the previous evening and that he couldn't remember the last time he slept so well.

On day 3 he hadn't needed pain medication since day 1. His wife was complaining about his snoring, that he was sleeping like a baby.

On day 4 he was pain free.

Six weeks on he is still pain free and off ALL his medication after being on paracetamol on a daily basis for years. Brings a smile to my face every time I think about it :)

POST ACCIDENT

"Today I had the most amazing result so far. I have been treating this woman who had the 8 car accidents. She has tried everything to make her pain go away for the past 3 years. She has generalized chronic pain with an intensity of 8/10 day and night. She has had chiropractic work every week, acupuncture, massage, reiki, physical therapy, injection therapy, heavy duty medication, she has consulted MD's, neurologist and nothing helped her, her chiropractor even told her he will pay the person who would be able to help her because he is out of resources right now. Her MD told her that she will never get better but worst with time and that she would age faster. Whatever all this people have said, believe it or not, this woman is actually pain free for the first time since 3 years. She just has stiffness over her neck on the left side. This is so crazy!!! I just can't believe it myself."

Healing the incurable

Raynaud's condition - Life is full of wonder!!!

Zoran.... 30 minutes ago I just worked on my wife's Raynaud's condition. One session for that condition. And guess what? She was working under some ice cold water afterwards (a sure no-no for years) and her fingers did not go numb and white! You know, I am still a little astonished. It's like being a kid again. I do not have answers. Life is full of wonder. The way it should be. :) Best thing I ever did was get out of the Answer Business!!!! :)

Well, I know you are busy. I am just pleased. :) :) And appreciative. Wanted to let you know.

Heart

Blood Pressure success

Just wanted to share a success story with high blood pressure. My husband's blood pressure had been super high for years, as high as 190/120 at times. It has taken about 4 months to get it down to normal, but I'm happy to say it's now down to 120/80 most of the time. … He was on as many as 7 or 8 medications at one point in time, and now we have reduced it to one quarter of one pill. It's probably another week before he believes enough to let go of that little shred of "modern medicine" but we'll get there!

Heart Arrhythmia result

"I had one 4 day treatment of BioEnergy healing which focussed on my heart, as I was experiencing over beating and had seen a cardiologist about it. I was given a monitor to wear for 24 hours and also an echo-scan, but the results took a long time to come through and, in the meantime, I contacted a Bioenergy Therapist. After day 3 of the treatment my heart normalised and I was thrilled. This was about a month ago now, and I still have status quo. I have seen my cardiologist again, and he has signed me off!"

Migraine

MIGRAINE

"I am experiencing amazing results using this method. I worked on a woman that was having hemiplegic migraines and in only one session she was headache free and her paralysis was gone after having the migraine since May of this year. The session was delivered a week after the level 1 seminar. She has been under the care of a neurologist for 2 years."

Severe Migraine Success

I had my first Migraine Patient last week.

This poor lady has been suffering with severe Migraine for 40 yrs! With dreadful head pain along with painful stabbing sensations in her left eye from the Migraine. After just 1 session, she said her pain levels had dropped from 8/10 to 1/10 and the stabbing pain in her left eye dissipated completely!

She was delighted and amazed by this result and I was almost speechless myself.

It is such an incredible joy to see real life results for real life problems with Bioenergy Therapy.

Neuromuscular

Alzheimer's patient - more alert and talking

email from a daughter after 1 four days treatment for her mom with Alzheimer's, June 3. 2012

Also, I visited my mom today - and my sister visited her yesterday. We both noticed the same thing - she is more alert than she has been - and happier - talking more, trying to communicate more, and she was even eating by herself using both hands when I came to visit her which is something she hasn't done before - she always needed the assistance of the nurses. So I think the healing sessions were helpful to her. I am looking forward to seeing what happens next! Thank you again!

ALS since 1995

"There have been significant observable improvements in my health since working with you (Z. H. Bioenergy Life Center). My swallowing has improved dramatically. My breathing at night has become easier. A growth on the top of my head has disappeared with only a slight trace. I sleep deeper with less out of control spasms. I have greater endurance on arm/leg aerobic exercise machine. I am a little stronger with weightlifting."

MS client - arm working again

"I have been working with a woman with advanced MS for a number of months. She has had little break troughs … lots of reduction of meds, etc. etc. But, she called me all excited on Saturday, saying "I had to share this with you… my left arm started working again, today!!!!!! I am so thrilled!!" She has been without the use of this arm for anything for more than a year."

B. has had MS for 10 years. He had one 20 - 30 minute treatment for 4 consecutive days

" …When B. arrived he could barely walk, and needed crutches. His right leg was stiff at the knee and affected the rest of the leg; we measured almost 3 inches of difference in length. He told me he couldn't walk up 10 steps to his mother's part of the house without holding on to the railing and using his other hand to drag up his leg. His healthy leg was stone cold, very bad circulation, his fingertips were tingling and the index finger on his left hand was also stone cold and not really flexible anymore, it got stuck at times, especially in the mornings just after waking up,.. he couldn't tie his shoe laces etc.

After the first session he went home walked up the stairs without helping along his leg, his toes didn't flex anymore. He called me up straight away and l thought he called because he forgot his crutches since he didn't even realize that he walked out without them…

Also his affected finger got flexibility and the leg is now just missing 1 cm to be back to the same length than his other leg, circulation has improved drastically, he can feel his leg again…Two days after his treatments were finished he had a MRT scan and found that MS is not progressing anymore. The doctor was stunned … for me (the therapist) it was amazing. "

MS - MRI scan shows 6 lesions gone

A wonderful MS result- Zoran just received a phone call from his client who has MS. After 8 treatments, one in person and the rest long distance, 6 lesions have disappeared according to her MRI – Purebioenergy was the only therapy she is doing and she is committed to it. Her doctor is surprised but told her to definitely continue so again, proof is in the results...

"Just wanted to let you know the results of my most recent MRI. I had an appointment with my neurologist yesterday and the results of my MRI showed that 6 Lesions in my brain have completely DISAPPEARED!!!!!! The Dr. says "whatever you are doing, keep doing it!"

Feeling better every week and continuing to improve. Thank you for doing this awesome work!!!"

V. R.April 25th 2012

Parkinson's client progress

J. and I have been working together for a little over a year to try to help his Parkinson's. He comes for treatments once a month for four consecutive days at a time. The Parkinson's hasn't gone away, but he has experienced significant improvement in his ability to function in daily life. For example, before starting the treatments, his tremor prevented him from typing after the effects of the last pills of the day had worn off in the evening, around 8:00 p.m. He's now able to type until he's ready for bed, around 11:00. He used to have a lot of trouble brushing his teeth, but that is no longer a problem. He can eat his Cheerios without their flying all over his apartment. Previously, he had to lay out everything in his apartment the night before, because he had a great deal of difficulty navigating when he first got up, but now he's able to get out of bed and move around without elaborate preparation. His general functioning has become much more even, without the extreme ups and downs that used to occur between the times when his pills were at their maximum and minimum effectiveness. At one point, his neurologist noticed that his walking had improved, and he decided that that was a good time to tell her about our treatments. She replied, "Well, it can't do any harm, and if you think it's helping, continue." ... J. definitely feel it's worth continuing the treatments at this point.

Parkinson's client - 57 yrs old - great response to Bioenergy

R., 57, was diagnosed with Parkinson's in 2007. He experienced difficulty with movement in general and with writing in particular and this caused him to give up his job. His energy levels were low. He had never experienced any energy therapy before and, although not a real skeptic, had doubts about whether a condition like Parkinson's would respond to anything like this. He is taking conventional medication and has had some problems with side effects and tolerance.

"Overall, I have had improvement in my mobility and balance. It is easier to move around and walking is easier. My general mobility is better and I am less slow, and this is reflected in finding it easier to get dressed and undressed, put my jacket on, and turn over in bed. I feel that my general energy levels are better than before treatment. The therapist noticed that my posture was much more upright, that I had lost the "Parkinson's stoop". I haven't monitored my posture myself, but this may help to explain why my balance and mobility are better. While being treated, I experienced strong feelings of heat when the therapist laid her hands on, for instance, my painful shoulder. I also at times felt tingling sensations moving down my spine...I feel that I have had an improvement in my general quality of life and I plan to have more treatment."

Stroke client - no more pain - hump on back reduced, hand opening, walking and cooking

Here is a daughter's report on mum's healing:

"Before my mum came to see you she used to look really dead and sad and just had no life in her. About 14 years ago she had a stroke on the left side of her brain and it affected all her right side of her body, her right hand and her speech. My mum finds it hard to use her hand and it used to just hang down by her side. We tried to get her to move it but she just couldn't move it at all. She grew this hump on her back and it used to cause her so much pain she would even walk bent over because of it. She was always saying her body was sore all the time. On the first day after seeing you my mum said that she was feeling really good and her head was not hurting like it use to. After her second visit she said that her thinking was clear and the lump on her back had come down heaps and she was standing up a lot more than before. I also noticed that she was using her right hand more and she could open it all the way up. By the 3rd and the 4th time coming to see you I noticed a BIG difference in her, the bump had gone and my mum was standing straight and honestly I had not seen her stand straight in a very long time. My mum would sit in her house and she never wanted to go out and would just stay home all the time. Now she is walking everywhere and sometimes twice a day. She now has more motivation to do things. She is even cooking which she didn't used to do. I am a great believer that you have healed my mum with your Bioenergy Therapy. It is amazing."

Stroke Recovery

Helping stroke in four days...

"I started treating a 67 year old lady that had a stroke 3 years ago. She liked the therapy right away and after the day 4 something amazing happened: she was able to straighten her right leg and put it on the chair.

Also...her right fist was opened,- it's been always closed and bent inwards since the stroke.

Since 2 weeks ago, sometimes fist is opened and sometimes closed.

I don't know if this can be consider a big improvement, but I think is is a HUGE improvement in such a short time.

After second round of therapy she is now able to say : "How are you" almost perfectly. Before we started therapy, she was only able to say that like a 2 year old.

Her husband told me that her right fist opens and closes (not when she wants it yet, but on it's own will), and her right leg is much straighter, and that she has LOTS of energy. Even when they walk, she now walks faster, he said that she almost runs."

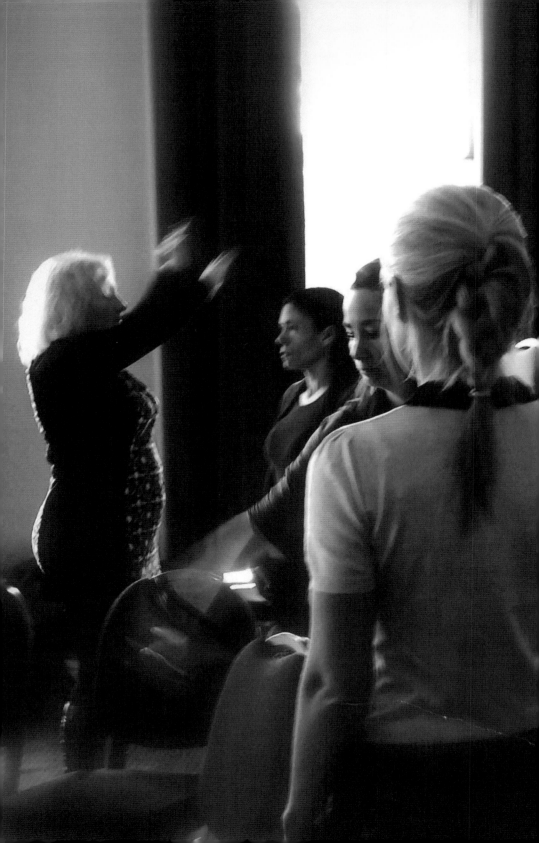

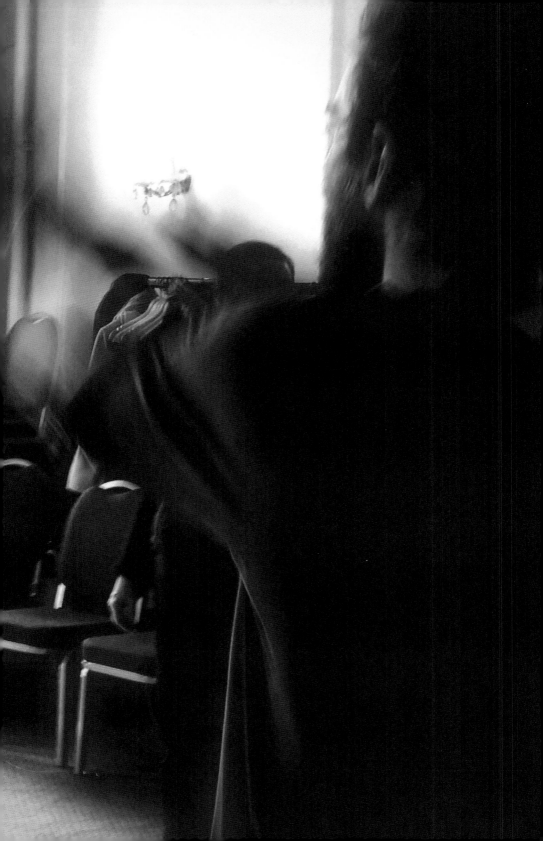

Respiratory Problems

Asthma - Mom and Dad

"So my wife and I attended level one and our first real health issue we have worked on is my youngest son and his asthma. Now before we started his treatment he was using his asthma inhaler multiple times each day. Literally after his 4th treatment, within minutes, his wheezing stopped altogether and he has not used his inhaler since.... it has been over a week. I have to say I am truly humbled to be able to be apart of his healing process. This has been an ongoing issue since he was a toddler. A big thank you to Zoran for teaching us this life changing method of healing."

Emphysema, bad circulation and ulcers on feet

Today I completed the therapy a client with emphysema, bad circulation and ulcers on feet. (He is also recovering from a stroke.) These are the results he's had so far:

1. Back pain diminished (only slight stiffness remains). Client staggered in my door a cripple and walked out with a smile on his face, limbs outstretched with a bit of a spring in his step.

2. When a nurse came to his house to dress the ulcers on his feet on day 2 of the treatment she noted that they were drying (he's had them for 3 years). Looking forward to find out what they will look like in a week!

3. When I asked him about his breathing (emphysema) on day 2 and 4 he only then realized he hadn't used his oxygen on those nights and had in fact forgotten about it. Before his first treatment he came in the door coughing, spluttering and wheezing and his chest was rattling and sounded hollow. When he left on the last day his breathing was relaxed and inaudible. He was actually singing as he left!

Skin

Burn wounds heal after 4 yrs

I started working last Thursday on a woman who had burned her feet and leg in 2009 with boiling oil. When she came to me she had limited movement, open bleeding sores and two toes that were starting to change colour. By Sunday she was moving her toes and all of the open wounds were closed. Her two toes were starting to change colour to a healthier pink. ... Just wish I had taken photos!

Eczema success

I have a friend who suffered severe eczema all over her body, which slowly got worse since January. Most of her face was inflamed, bleeding here and there, feeling itchy everywhere. When she came for the treatment it was shocking to see how much she's suffering...Even after a first day she felt so much better, her face started to recover and not feeling itchy, energy level increased, she said she could finally do something and not just sit and suffer. I was so happy for her, it was amazing - such a difference on her face from inflamed to calming down each day ending up very significantly recovered - if I could just show you, it was like 80% recovered in 4 days! That's awesome!

The other day she came for a 2 session of 4 days having a break of 10 days in between and she said she had no more eczema on her body. Her face returned to normal, just a slight staining and skin feeling tight on her face, she said everyday has been some improvement. We started new sessions and she feels even more relief. It's great to be able to help in such a simple way.

10 year old girl with excellent facial eczema result

The 10 year old client no longer feels she has to wear sunglasses to stop people staring at the red eczema around her eyes. She even stood up in front of her whole class and gave a presentation without her sunglasses on. Sunglasses are now worn as sunglasses rather than a means of hiding her eyes. Joy of joys :-)

Skin Rash (distant healing)

A man who had spent several days in the Belizean jungle (Central America) called me to say that a skin rash broke out on his face several days after returning to the States. The rash was not responding to anything he had taken internally or applied topically. He stated that the itching became so intense that, in his words, "I literally wanted to scratch my face off."

He actually went to an emergency room the night before he called to see if they would give him an injection of morphine!

He heard about Bioenergy from a mutual friend and decided to try it. I followed the protocol for "Psychogenic Illnesses". When he called me the day of his 2nd session, he said, "I can't believe this! I expected to feel a little better after the 4 day session, but I already feel 95% better after only the first session!" He was truly amazed.

He continued to improve … I have spoken to him since then, and the rash has not returned.

Sports Injuries

Athlete leg injury

Mom's story about her athletic daughter's long distance therapy success.

My daughter is an athlete who fences five to six days a week and also runs about 5-10 miles a day. In the spring, she injured her leg and couldn't walk or put any pressure on it. We took her to see an orthopedic doctor who x-rayed her leg and told us that there were no breaks or fractures. He told us it was probably a bruised tendon and that she could wear an orthopedic boot to help speed the healing and that she would not be able to run or fence until her leg healed. We waited two months, and her leg didn't get better; she still had the same level of pain. Discouraged, I researched various options and came across a video called, Think About It, by Zoran Hochstatter. … why not try the Bioenergy Healing method? What did we have to lose? I talked to my daughter about this method … and to my surprise, she actually wanted to try this. I think part of her openness was because she felt discouraged by the previous medical approach.

I contacted Zoran Hochstatter and asked if he was available to treat her and if it was possible to do this, since he was in Europe and we were in the United States. Zoran assured me he could do this remotely. We decided to go ahead and try this method and on the first day of my daughter's therapy, I knew that this was not like anything we have ever experienced.

Zoran asked her what her pain level was: from a level 1 to 10 (with 10 being the most painful and current state of pain she was in). After the twenty minute therapy, he called her back and … the pain level was now at level 7. She could now put pressure on her leg and walk with much less pain. And when she later described her experience to me, I think I was more surprised than she was. She told me that she felt a wave going through her body, warmth at the site of her injured leg, bubbling beneath the skin where her injury was, and tingling throughout her body. On the final day of her therapy, my daughter's pain level was now zero.

The next day, my daughter went back to fencing and ran five miles. The healing was whole, complete and permanent; there was no return of pain. I am writing this three months later and she continues to fence and run without any pain.

Gymnast's Leg injury healed

BACKGROUND OF THE PROBLEM: My daughter (former Jr. Olympian in gymnastics) tore her ACL and had it repaired by Surgical Graft back in December. (I had not taken level 1 at that time).

Fast forward 3 months: She has been living away, at college since the surgery. She was having problems in post-op healing. Significant pain. Could not bend her knee past 40 degrees. Walked with a stiff leg. Please note: She had been getting Physical Therapy twice per week for more than 3 months. And this was all the progress they had made.

PROTOCOL: I got her to come home from college 4 days early for her appointment with the surgeon to check on her progress. I did one (1) Treatment. Wellness plus warmed the knee. That was all. (She was moving better on the 4th day, but the Doctor said she might need to go back under the knife. He was not happy with her progress.)

1O DAYS LATER: Dramatic Improvements. #1 NO PAIN!!! #2. Her range of motion more than DOUBLED in less than 2 weeks! She can ride a bike again! And she does not walk with a limp!!

I was happy. She was ecstatic! No more surgery needed!

Stress/Anxiety/Psychogenic

Bi Polar

"I recently worked with a gentleman who was diagnosed with Bi Polar disorder when he was 14 or so. Lithium seemed to stabilise him more than anything else. About 6 months ago he was told by his doctor that he could not continue to use Lithium on account of the apparent damage it had caused to his liver and kidneys – he's in his mid 40's now. Since the change in medication he had been hospitalised 7 times for bi polar episodes, and was despairing his future. He told his psychiatrist that he wanted to work with me, and 3 weeks ago we worked away over the 4 days. The following week his psychiatrist was impressed enough to allow him return to work and certified that he is fit to drive again. My client certainly did say he was feeling stronger in himself, more positive and more energised. …Although there's no guarantee that he won't have another BPD episode, I have to say, of all of the recent work that I have done this was one of the more satisfying cases, because he really did seem to have suffered with BPD for so long and at a lot of personal cost to him…

I hope this helps someone else out there who may suffer from, or know someone who suffers from BPD."

Costochondritis Healing

I suffered Costochondritis for over 10 years. I was treated with the anxiety protocol and received a profound healing! Prior to healing I was unable to wear a bra except for the most extreme circumstances, this inhibited my ability to attend a great deal of things, events, and social situations. I was rushed by ambulance to the ER last March because it became so constricting that I could not breath. I was hyperventilating and suffocating at the same time. It was after that episode that I sought out Bioenergy healing. I now wear a bra with ease and my life has opened up tremendously. I have so many stories to share about what bioenergy has done for me, this is only one area of healing.

Depression Success Story

From a client with Depression

"I cannot tell you, Z., how much better I feel after having the therapy with you. I have not had an incident of depression since…I don't think I could get depressed even if I tried. This has set my life in a different course."

Sister diagnosed with psychosis/schizophrenia

Hi there,

Well, there is good news about W. Her speech is continuing to improve, her energy is absolutely on the mend. She says she's starting to get an interest in things again. She has described herself as an elastic band that snapped but she can feel herself bouncing back.

She has an appointment with the psychiatrist on Monday and her husband has promised her that he won't let the doctor put her back on the injections for the psychosis/schizophrenia.

She has been really good in this respect and last night was the first time that I've been talking to her that she hasn't mentioned anything unusual.

She did say a few weeks ago that the was going to watch what she said in front of people as she didn't want to go back on the medication. She is very anti drugs.

So it is a little difficult to assess it fully but I (and everyone else) believe that she is so, so much better.

She also has talked about being embarrassed about running of to different countries to crack the code but at least she is talking about it. She has also expressed fears about a number of things. Perhaps you could help her with that??

The ripple effect has been amazing, my mother is sleeping again, her husband is the happiest he's been in years, her kids are getting their mother back, W. is thankful everyday for her second chance, it's fabulous. Thank you so much.

I will let you know how the doctor appointment goes on Monday?

Cheers

Hi there,

W. had her appointment today and the doctor is happy for her to continue without medication. Happy days!!!

Plenty of sleep at last

Was delighted to begin using my new healing skills the day after leaving St. Petersburg training! Worked with a friend and her insomnia with very happy results. She is getting lotzzzzzzzzzz of sleep now. And she says "...finding that sleep is wonderful! Even if I wake in the night I can get back to sleep" So happy for her!

PTSD - former Marine

Testimony from a Former Marine from the first Gulf war. Has a medical record noting exposure to nerve agent.

"I was diagnosed with PTSD, had lung issues, messed up ankle from a bad service related injury, bad knees, my lower back all the way to my neck and left shoulder were in constant pain. I was diagnosed by the Veterans hospital with a sleep disorder, and couldn't sleep more than a couple hours and the quality of the sleep was really bad.. I was extremely angry and lived on the edge of feeling suicidal or homicidal on any given day. I had a bioenergy treatment and by the end of the first one I could finally get some sleep. Most of the pain in my body went away on the first couple days, a lot of the injuries are really old. My ankle doesn't hurt anymore and it has been giving me problems for 20 yrs. I feel less aggression, and I'm not depressed or suicidal and Not angry. Ive been sleeping every night so far and the results have been great. I feel a lot better. I am coming to the class in the DC area to learn how to do this."

Bio Energy Therapy brings REAL Relief for PTSD Victims

PTSD, (Post Traumatic Stress Disorder), is not just a problem for military veterans but also for victims of sexual assault, domestic violence and other crimes, along with survivors of severe accidents and acute life-threatening illness.

Over the past several months I have had the opportunity to provide

PUREBIOENERGY (an energy healing modality) for many clients, both civilian and military with a diagnosis of PTSD. As these clients have been undergoing Bioenergy Therapy I've not only watched them evolve back into a normal, functioning, and healthy life; but I've witnessed a revolution in their thinking and a total evolution in their recovery impacting not only themselves, but also their much appreciative families.

Real Relief

Purebioenergy healing has been an effective form of real relief for a large and growing number of people suffering with a diagnosis that has left the military medical system drowning in case loads and with little resources to answer this challenge.

In the military medical community PTSD has been described as a "growing epidemic". With fiscal constraints of the government looming, Bioenergy Therapy provides a safe, low cost and measurable results based treatment, and it's not medicine.

It's an alternative to the old solution of counseling and medication; which the medical community and clients with this diagnosis have expressed their own frustration. This frustration is due to a lack of real healing or results from conventional methods.

How do you know if someone you love has PTSD?

Common symptoms of PTSD are:

- Frequent Nightmares
- Re-occurring memories of a traumatic event
- Sleeplessness or difficulty sleeping
- Feeling on edge, anxiety or panic attacks
- Jumpy at the sound of sudden noises
- Anger and irritability
- Lost interest in family, life and past interests
- Trouble keeping focused on one subject
- Difficulty relating to friends and family
- Increase in usage of drugs and/or alcohol as a coping mechanism

Common complaints amongst Veterans who have tried counseling or "talk therapy" is that they don't want to continue to relive the pain and trauma over and over again in group therapy or private sessions. One Veteran stated that he felt "worse" after he attended the counseling. Another Veteran said medication made him feel disconnected, numb and groggy and destroyed his ability to be intimate with his wife.

The answer is much Simpler.

Bioenergy Therapists work only with pure energy from the Source. This energy contains intelligence and the blue print to health that your immune system needs to strengthen and reverse any condition or illness within the body.

There is no reliving of trauma over and over again in order to bring PTSD victims relief. The client sits comfortably in a chair for about 15 minutes and the Bioenergy Therapist does a few specific moves.

No Side Effects with Bioenergy Therapy… except for an increased feeling of wellness and a refocusing of the immune system to elevate pain and promote healing within the body.

On this journey I've met many people desperate for help with PTSD and often they feel they are out of options for relief. I have come to understand just how much Bioenergy Therapy has changed the lives affected by PTSD.

Surgery

Hernia disappears and no surgery needed…

Someone just came to me this week for hernia - after they saw the doctor and were told that they had to have surgery, again. She then came to me to see if Bioenergy could work before going through another surgery. After the first session she had no pain and the hernia disappeared. She did all 4 sessions - and there is no trace of the hernia. It appears that hernias can be treated by Bioenergy methods.

Hip Operation Client

87 year old N. was in hospital for hip operation, then had complica-

tions and ended up in hospital with kidney failure. His blood sugar level was high, he was unresponsive, and doctor's prognosis was grim.

His wife called me, and I did a long distance treatment. She observed that he was calm, and smiling during treatments. His leg (operated) would move, and also his arms. On the 3rd day he was eating, and sitting up. I also did a treatment for S (his wife), because she was tired, physically & mentally. After the first day she was able to sleep, and had more energy. With every day she was feeling more calm, and stronger.

After 15 days she informed me that her husband talks a lot more and looks much better. His blood and urine analysis were good as well as his vitals and blood sugar levels.

Then, a week ago, she asked me for more treatments because he had trouble getting up due to painful inflamed joints. I did 3 days so far (in person), tomorrow is the last day, but there is huge improvement already.

Today I received this email from his wife:

"I have noticed a marked improvement in N's walking and getting up from the bed and chairs

He looks better - - more healthy, almost like before the accident.

His feet and joints are not swollen as they were previous to your treatment.

His appetite is a lot better.

His spirit is much better during the day."

Using Purebioenergy at home, a husband's story....

"I just had surgery 3 days ago to reattach the pectoral tendon and have been taking a lot of pain medication to keep the pain in check. My wife did a therapy session on me last night before I went to bed. I woke up this morning with very little pain and have not needed to take any pain meds today. That is amazing to say the least considering how much pain I have been in since the surgery. I am very interested to see how rapidly I heal now with bioenergy therapy!

Just to follow up I have not needed pain meds since my wife started the sessions. I wonder how my doctor will explain this!"

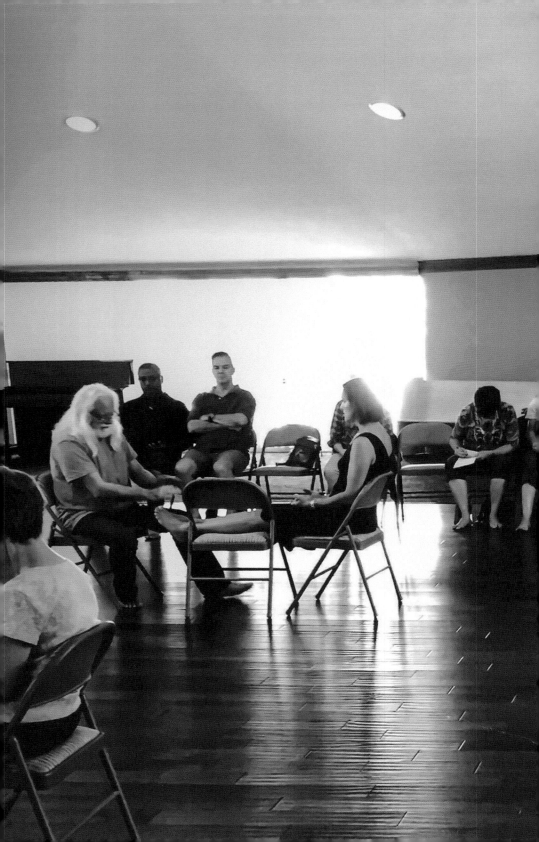

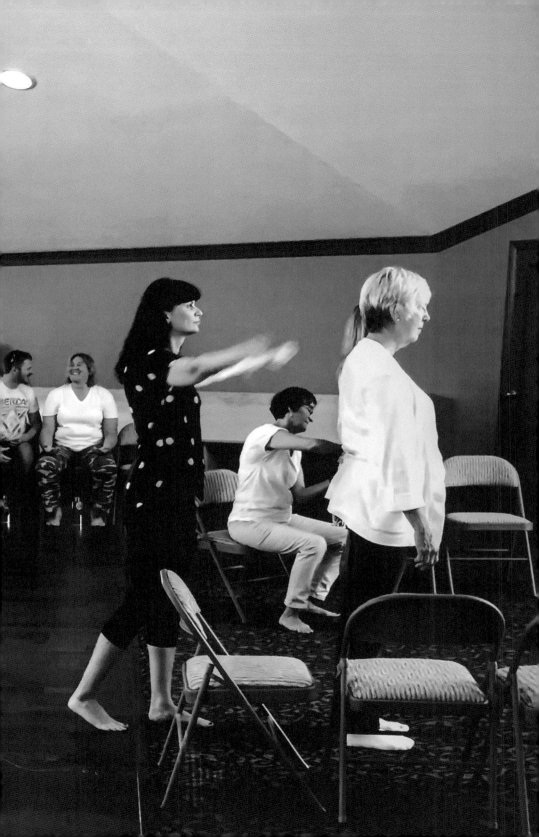

Varicose Veins

Bad veins and Blood clots

"I recently had a long distance client with bad veins and blood clots. I did the varicose vein protocol and warming where the blood clots were. The problem resolved in 4 days completely. No more blood clots and no more painful and burning legs :)"

Viruses

Hep C

I treated a woman diagnosed with Hepatitis C at the beginning of December '08. When she was first diagnosed in 2003, her viral load (measures the amount of hepatitis in the blood) was 8 million. In October '08 her viral load was up to 17.6 million. She went back for another test 10 days after her first therapy with me (2 months after her October results) and was very pleased to learn her viral load had dropped to 5.4 million. Her M.D. made no comment after looking at the recent results.

She has never taken any medication for Hep-C, and the only thing she's done differently since October '08 was the 4-day Bioenergy Therapy. We just completed her second 4-day therapy this afternoon.

Herpes

"...thank you for helping me with a chronic herpes condition which has plagued my life for over 15 years. It took a couple of session to see results, but I knew I had to stick with it. By session 3-4 I started seeing much less outbreaks, something that was happening 70-80% of the time. By session 6 the change was pretty drastic. We have done 8 sessions together and at this point I can eat anything and there is no outbreak.

...By far, this method will reverse any condition - I completely know it! Herpes creates such a stigma in our society and is labeled "incurable", that words cannot express what means to regain back my health and my freedom. I now KNOW that every condition is reversible! Thank you for helping me regain my life back!"

HIV/AIDS - Freddie's story

Here's Freddie's story, condensed into a paragraph, minus all the remarkable physical changes, tear jerking details, and praises from both his parents crediting me with saving the life of their son (although I know it was the method that created the optimal environment for him to heal himself).

"Freddie's CD4 count was 179 when we began his first 4-day session (below 200 is classified as AIDS). One week later it was up to 400. After a second 4-day session it increased to 563 and his viral load was down to 75. His doctor said, "You can't get much better than 75." Five MONTHS later his CD4 was above 700 and his viral load was "virtually non-existent." His doctor said that in his 25 years of treat-ing AIDS patients, Freddie went from being the worst case he's ever seen to making the most dramatic improvement he's ever seen."

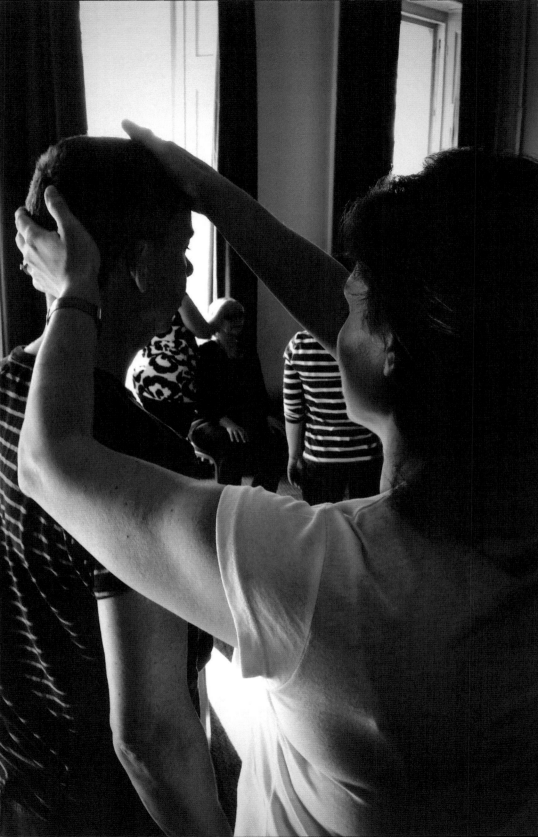

user friendly

Therapy with Bioenergy is any therapy using the same energy.

Working with it, or manipulating Bioenergy can be intuitive, frustrating, painful, hard to perform, mysterious, or structured, simple and easy.

This book talks primarily about the of use Bioenergy in its purest way, which makes it structured, simple, easy to learn and easy to use.

The energy is pure, when it does not contain any pollutants of your own thinking.

Once your craft of manipulating the Bioenergy is on autopilot, the knowledge of techniques was absorbed, you "stop thinking" and everything happens automatically.

When the energy is applied correctly it is user friendly for the therapist and for the client. The techniques are simple and precise. They are stripped of all the nonsense and what's left is packed with purpose and functionality.

Each technique has a defined function and, at the same time, has other purposes as well, reaching into deep, complex layers of this ancient wisdom.

Each particular technique, while delivering information with a healing effect for the client is also, at the same time, protecting the healer.

green is in

Most of our activities burn some kind of energy. Most of the time it stems from a non-renewable, finite source, be it food for us or gas for our car. We use it up, and it is gone.

There is always a byproduct of that used energy. A pollutant, be it methane from our food exiting our exhaust, or some other gas exiting some pipe or the other.

Using Bioenergy, on the other hand, is clean. It being a creative thought energy, it does not physically pollute the environment. It means we have a choice, because we do.

Not believing in choices is a sign of thinking with somebody else's head. It means believing what we were told we must believe. So now we believe that we need oil for our transportation. We believe that our health cannot change for the better without pharmaceuticals or, at least, we have to have some doctor, even if he is only a chiropractor, agree with a different solution. And when the shit really hits the fan we usually go for the worst solution that killed many people before.

Creative thought energy can be incredibly polluting and the best proof for this is the state of our civilization. It is the result of the present, ongoing, old paradigm. Greed, wars, hunger, illness and misery are results of what we think about ourselves, and about the priorities of our existence.

Well, then, you can argue that physical pollution comes from our way of thinking, and it does. But if we start thinking differently, if we start seeing possibilities of different choices, if we start thinking with our own head, we can surely break this chain of conditioning which enslaves us.

Repeating the thoughts we were served from the moment we were born, confusing them with knowledge, we are paralyzed in our helplessness even though the solution is simple: think with your own head. Think your thoughts and gain knowledge by direct, first hand experience.

Only you can clean your mind. Practice mental hygiene like you practice physical cleanliness.

How are we going to prevent pollution? Who is polluting? You are.

Watch what you think and make it green.

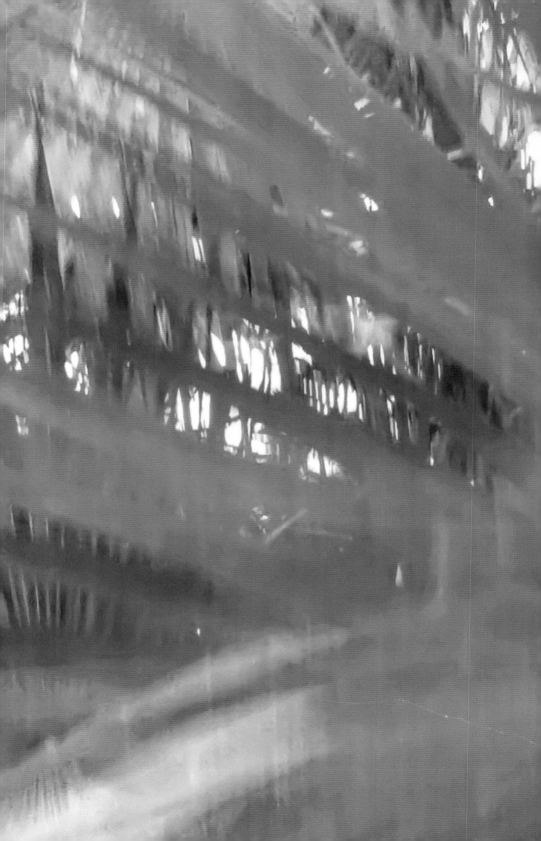

THOUGHTS ABOUT BIOENERGY

BIOENERGY is not energy needed as body fuel for the functioning of the body. Every organ and every cell uses energy for its many functions. They use chemical energy in the form of ATP molecules.

BIO PHOTONS are also not Bioenergy. They are electromagnetic frequencies emitted by all living organisms and are possibly a part of communication system between cells.

IN EUROPE, the term bioenergy is also used for renewable energy produced from biological sources. In the US, the term biofuel is used instead.

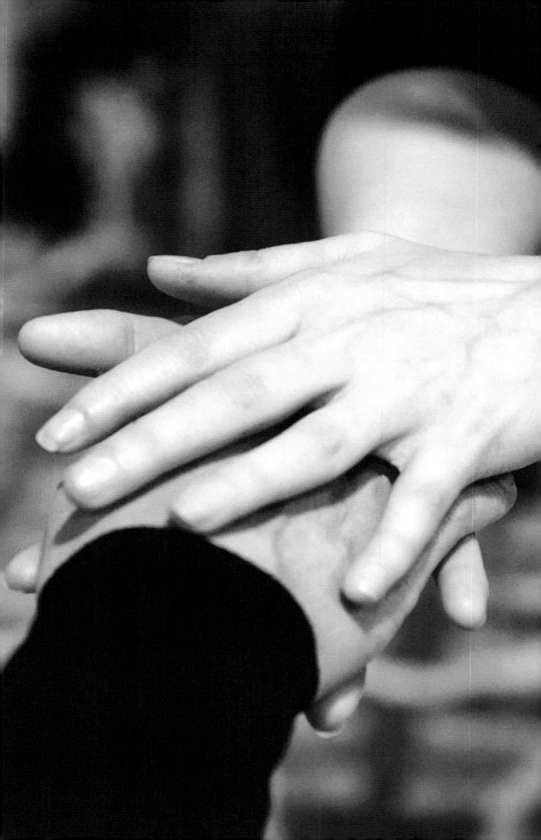

help your mother

Maybe this is the way to pay your mother back. Even if your mother caused you harm in some way, and they all did, she did it with the best intention and that entitles her to some payback.

Most of us love our mothers and it is even better when we can do something for them.

- Is she in pain?

- Is she forgetting more than she should?

- Is she depressed (or just grumpy)?

- Is she old and needs a little energy boost?

- Is she overmedicated and foggy?

You can help your mom with all these problems. Even if you don't address her cancer, by applying pure Bioenergy, you will make her life noticeably better.

Don't forget to remove yourself from the healing process. Even though "mother knows best" make sure that she trusts the fact that YOU can help her. You have to work harder to earn her trust and even though it will seem that you are doing less, caring less, stay on that "beach" with total belief in your capabilities.

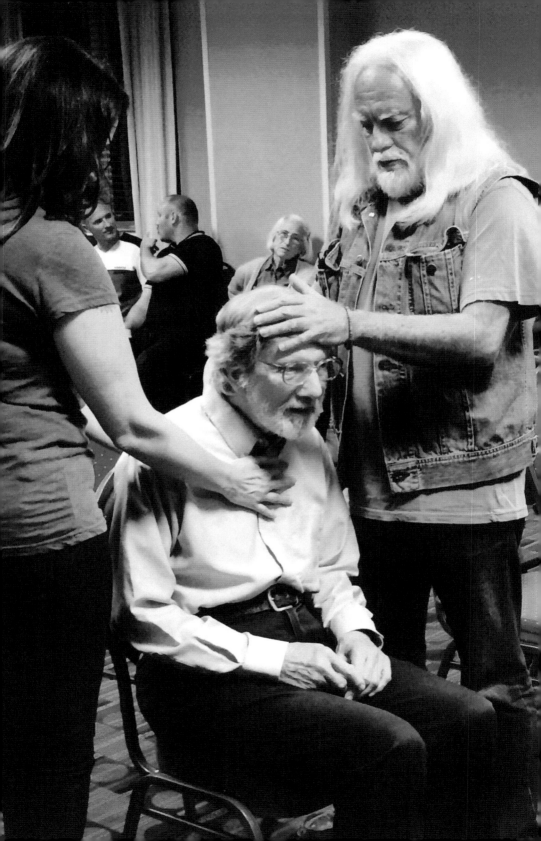

help
your father

Your father has problems with his prostate. Or he is fighting dementia. Maybe he is just simply depressed after his retirement. He can't enjoy his hobby as he used to.

When we apply the Bioenergy in its purest form we don't just eliminate the physical problem. We reach them on the subconscious level, where most of our decisions are made, and cause the transformation of the way they think and act.

Seniors

80 yr old runs up the stairs

An old lady, about 80 years old, has for many, many years had problems with her joints in both shoulders and legs.

Doctors told her that this is arthropathy and "this is how it is to be old - you have to live with it". Since her daughter is very receptive to bioenergy healing, she wanted to just try it. We decided to do it Long Distance.

Now 10 days after the treatment she called me and said she is almost running up stairs as she did when she was young - didn't think it was possible to feel that way again as an old lady.

She is so happy!

Now she´s heading for session no. 2 and is looking forward to what else can happen, and what can be done with her shoulder.

I feel such a grace towards this method. Life is full of meaning!

96 yr old - incontinence gone

My aunt who is 96 had one distance healing (4 sessions) and was totally cured from her incontinence after the first session. When I called her to follow up after 10 days her voice sounded strong, full and rich (due to her age her voice had become faint) and she told me not only was she very happy to have no more problems with in-continence but also felt so energetic and had done 30 sit-ups every day the last few days!!

Grandmother had a bad fall - full recovery after Bioenergy Therapy - Mother's anxiety gone

My grandmother had a bad fall… she was in Intensive Care Unit with brain hemorrhaging, a badly broken arm and her heart stopped at one point and they had to bring her back. My mother heard the news and she was having terrible anxiety and was on the verge of a panic attack she was so worried and upset - she let me work on her (this is HUGE - my mother is not a believer) and her anxiety went away after just one treatment and did not come back. I worked on my grandmother for four days and there were significant improvements, but most notably she had severe pain in her chest near her heart (she thought maybe they'd bruised one of her upper ribs when they resuscitated her) that made it so she couldn't breathe deeply, or cough or laugh or move around without grimacing. She said the pain was more severe than her broken arm. After the first Bioenergy treatment - that pain in her chest completely disappeared and did not return. She was amazed! She continues to improve every day and will make a full recovery. She turns 85 next week.

Well... that has been totally amazing!

Hi Zoran,

Well...... that has been totally amazing!

John was improved yesterday after a good night sleep but still slurring speech and the left side not co-operating.

I did the first session of the Stroke Protocol around noon. He could feel the "feet manipulation" and said it felt like "vibration".

After that he slept for 2 hours.

Since then he has been better than he has been in weeks. Sitting straighter, improved walking. Clear speech.

The droopy left side of mouth also entirely gone. Lots of witty comments and teasing the caregivers.

He ate his soup using his left hand with no signs of tremor!

The household has gone from extreme stress to absolute happiness.

It was like being in a time warp, as if the collapse (stroke symptoms) the previous day had not happened.

Many many thanks for your help. I feel that the healing started the moment I decided to email you for advice.

Big Hug!

Love Cathie

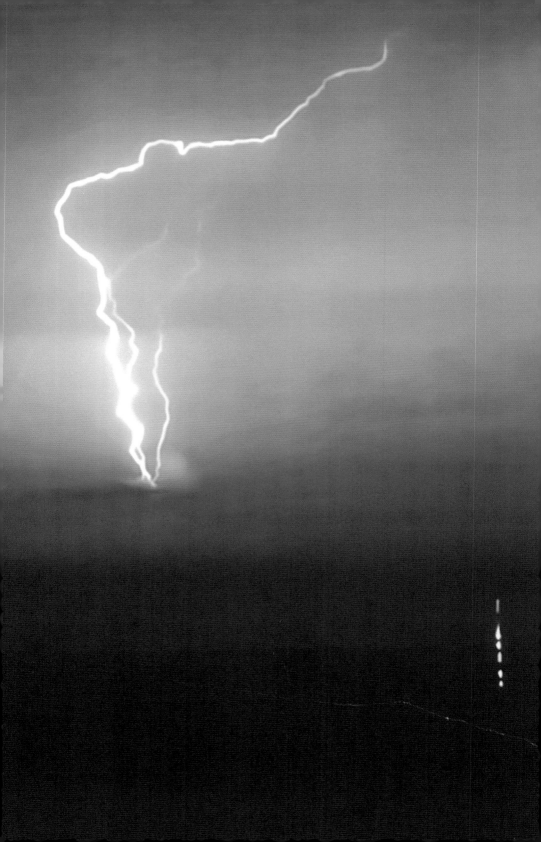

no harming side effects

Bioenergy, when applied correctly, cannot harm you. This energy is informed, intelligent and contains all the information your body needs. It is the "breath of life".

We can, then, say that the effect of it is life. Then the side effects manifest as living, growing, being happy, sad, loving, and everything in between.

It is amusing how Pharmaceutical companies talk about side effects of their drugs. Side effect is an effect. Period. Aftershock or a pre-shock is also an earthquake and will, if it is strong enough, kill you just as effectively as the main tremor.

The only (side)effect of Bioenergy is more life.

And then you die.

Well, as long as you die happy.

Medical professionals using the method

Review from Holistic Health Practitioner

Since taking the Bio-Energy course I have worked on a number of people. The results have been nothing short of miraculous. People I work on are absolutely shocked when after just 10 minutes of working on them their pain is completely eliminated. It is so wonderful to be able to help people in this way. I have been in the healing field for over 8 years and never have I done so much in so little time. This method is truly miraculous in nature. It defies what we presently understand about life. This energy field we live in and are supported by truly can be used to heal ourselves and those we love. Thanks so much for inviting me to this training and for your continued support as I spread my wings and become an even more effective healer.

Review by Dr. Carol Langley

Having been in chiropractic practice for 11 years, I put myself on a constant search for healing. My quest took me well beyond continuing education requirements. I found that there was no one technique which worked for everyone. I took pride in tailoring care to the person's needs, at that moment while they were in my presence. I trained in Reiki and eventually became a Reiki Master. I studied many chiropractic techniques, being drawn more to low force, less invasive touch, seeking to honor the person with whom I was working. About 3 years ago, my studies caused me to look above the spine to the cranium, which I now realize is essential for true "correction" to take place and for patterns to change permanently. Then, in June 2007, a blessing came to me in the form of Bioenergy

Healing, a method that is so simple, so in alignment with universal laws and life, that it may seem unbelievable to most people. Thankfully, this method has been brought to the United States via Zoran Hochstatter, and I was privileged to participate in one of the first training classes. Since learning Bioenergy, life has changed for the better. I feel even more confident that true healing is available to every person. Seemingly "permanent" or "incurable" conditions/diseases are clearing before our eyes, as is seen in the video ("Think About It"). You know that someone really has something when they can share the "how to" successfully with others. It's not just that they have a special "gift" since you quickly discover that you can do some of this "magical" healing work as well, immediately after training. I feel graciously honored to be a part of this revolutionary system of healing that the planet so desperately needs.

Dr. Carol Langley, D.C.

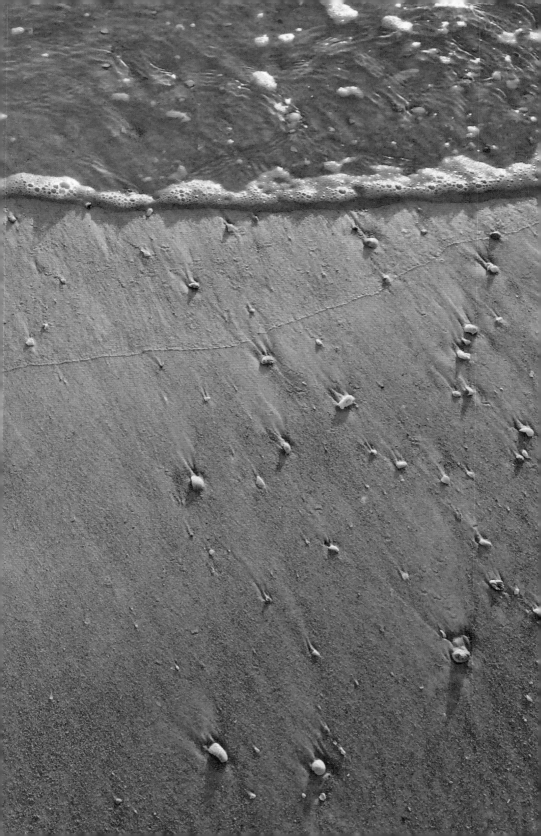

THOUGHTS ABOUT BIOENERGY

ENERGY WORK, in the purest sense of energy healing, occurs when the energy, with the information contained in it, causes the transformation necessary for the body to heal. The "frequency" itself is information, and the body understands this communication.

EVERYTHING is energy but not every segment of this "cosmic whole" is beneficial for us. In other words, when we separate frequencies from the whole, using only specific frequencies, we will get different effects and uses for them. Some will be practical and some will be downright destructive and deadly. Balance is the key.

THE PROBLEM arises when we think we know what we are using, when in fact we mostly misunderstand the word energy. There are different kinds of energy and for healing purposes we only use Bioenergy.

Distance Healing

BLADDER TUMOR GONE - LONG DISTANCE

Doctor is baffled about tumor– "It was there and now its gone?" Last week Zoran's relative was diagnosed with a bladder tumor…after one 4 day distance treatment the tumor was found to have disappeared by the perplexed oncologist. Needless to say she is very happy.

First long distance results — dancing in the kitchen

Right after level 2 in Seattle a few weeks ago I took the plunge and did Distance Healing….My brother who lives in Belgium, has never heard of bio energy…Having been in a lot of pain for over 15 years, following a car accident, and taking strong pain killers with less and less relief he was at the end of his rope. Out of desperation he asked for my help.

After the first treatment the pain dropped from a 10 to a 3. Everyday after that was exhilarating and by the end of the treatment he and his wife were speechless. The transformation was amazing…. she told me he was dancing in the kitchen ;)

In truth, the experiences of the past few weeks ~ the seminars and the practice of the method ~ have changed ME more than words can tell. I have no "gift". I do not see auras. I do not feel energy blockages in chakras. I thought I was doomed to watch the parade from the sidewalk. Today I feel I am in the parade and it is FUN!!!

Such a breakthrough… such life giving feeling.

A long distant healing from Florida to South Carolina

HIPS AND KNEES

"In February of 2010, I had my 5 year checkup on my hips. When I complained that my knees were hurting, my doctor took a series of x-rays of my knees. He told me that I was "bone on bone" in my knees and asked when did I want to schedule the replacement surgery. My response was "never".

After trying to cut my grass in March, I found that I couldn't finish the yard in one session. It usually took 1 hour and 15 minutes of straight walking. After 45 minutes I had to stop. I knew I had to do something to relieve the pain…so an old friend said she could help me out with that through Bioenenergy sessions. When she told me that she could do this over the phone, I was very skeptical. She gave me a web site and some information and told me to call her if I needed some help. After the 4 days of long distant bioenergy sessions I decided to try to cut my grass. With absolutely no pain, I buzzed through cutting the grass in a little less than the 75 minutes it usually took. I was very happy with the results. I had no pain, and standing for long periods of time was not a problem.

After about 5 weeks, I started to feel my knees tightening up. I thought that maybe another set of sessions…So, in the first week of June, we did another 4 sessions long distance. After these sessions, I was able to be pain free, to cut the grass in under an hour. This is during Columbia's hottest summer, when the temperature was 95+ with a heat index of 105. It's now the middle of October, four and half months later. I was able to attend the Columbia Blues Festival, 10/1-10/2, Friday night and all day Saturday, standing on my feet, dancing the day away, without pain.

It has been a great relief that I haven't had to visit my doctor in the past 10 months. I hope to stay with the program and stay away from the knife. Thank you very much."

Long Distance Results from a therapist who just finished a Level two seminar in NY

80 yr old delighted with LD result

I just finished the 4th day treatment. After surgery the client's pain was a 6, on 2nd day after surgery we did therapy and his pain went down to a 3. By the 3rd session he reported no pain or swelling at all. In fact he felt wonderful. Today he felt well and balanced and was so appreciative of the work. He's 80! And he's a doctor and energy worker. He was just delighted. I'm in DC , he's in California and he really felt it coming through. I am so grateful for this work.

Incredible energy work - instantaneous and lasting result

"Thank you, for the incredible energy work! My neck is dramatically improved, and my pain greatly diminished. The most astonishing aspect to me is that the long distance energy work was as powerful as the in-person hands on healing. I have tried many healing modalities, from conventional to alternative, but none provided such an instantaneous and lasting result as your energy healing. Thank you seems inadequate! "D.B. Westchester County, NY

Son treats mother for Sjogren's Disease

My mother was 85 when I started to treat her for Sjogren's syndrome.

(For the record, the personal reason I took Level 2, was so that I could treat her condition - it is considered to be unrecoverable, and typically the symptoms worsen and make the patient becomes more uncomfortable over time. This was her experience. I live more than a thousand miles away from her, so the best approach was to use the PureBioenergy Method in a "distance" setting.)

For more than a dozen years, she had continued to degrade and suffer from this disease. Sjogren's syndrome is an autoimmune disorder in which the glands that produce tears and saliva are destroyed. This causes dry mouth and dry eyes, very dry ear canals and other problems. The condition may affect other parts of the body, including the kidneys and lungs, but in her case, the most frustrating thing to her was she sounded stoned or drunk when she talked because she could not get her tongue and lips to unstick - and she had heavily slurred speech, her digestion was constantly having problems since digestion starts in the mouth with chewing and saliva.

She was on three different medications to make her more comfortable, including one to help her tears - when she blinked she felt like she had sand in her eyes. Not a fun way to age! (By the way, these symptoms were experienced WITH the medications she was taking to relieve the symptoms. They were not working well, at all!)

I started treating her as soon as finished level 2 training (Zoran gave me a protocol, since the condition was not "listed"). In addition to the Basic Wellness, we added eyes, ears, mouth, and positive therapy up the spine.

Every other week, I treated her, for about 6 months, with only a few weeks break in between. She wanted to stay at it because she was seeing small, but measurable progress.

6 months later, she was off all of her meds. She speaks clearly now - and get this - she can give anyone she wants - a big, wet, juicy, "raspberry"!! (Hey, if you are 85 or 86 and very feisty, this is a very important thing to be able to do!) Many, many thanks for the chance to do this for my own Mom!!

So, to those who say that Sjogren's is incurable, they can call my Mom and she will give them a raspberry! That should be all the proof they would need!

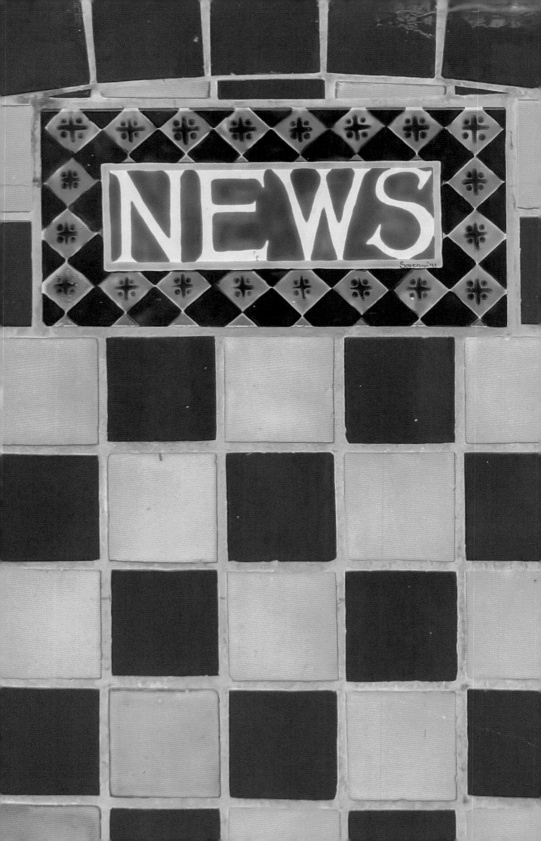

works on
every biofield

Our energy body, sometimes also called a biofield, is our matrix, a blueprint, our defense system; our immune system.

This is the universal healer in us that keeps us healthy. If our immune system does not function properly, we are sick. When our defense system is put back in order, and it assumes its function, the body heals.

We work with life itself streaming through our hands.

Can it get any better? Yes, in reality it can. It gets better when the person, which we work on, also accepts it without adding any of the conditioning that made him, or her, ill in the first place.

you
can help
your plants

Are we talking about your azalea plant
or your olive grove?
Your choice.
Bioenergy works on every living
thing, including plants. You can
make their fruits sweeter and
their flowers lusher.

Plants

Tree healing...

Did bioenergy treatment for a tree and got a cool update from a client.

Tree used to be beautiful, but when she moved it it seemed to get sick. When I came over to look at it, it had a lot of moss, mold, what looked like a tumor growing on it, but some leaf buds starting. Last year, it grew leaves that fell off shortly after they grew.

It's been a little over 2 weeks since I finished and she sent me this picture with a note that the tree was definitely doing better. Not only does it have leaves still, but it has bloomed too in a big way. So cool. :-)

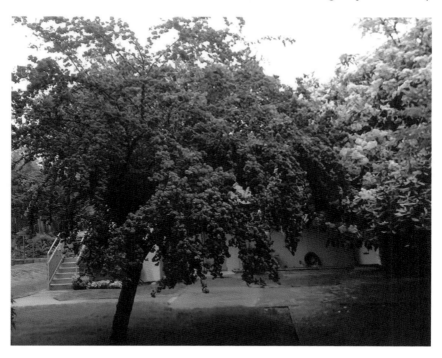

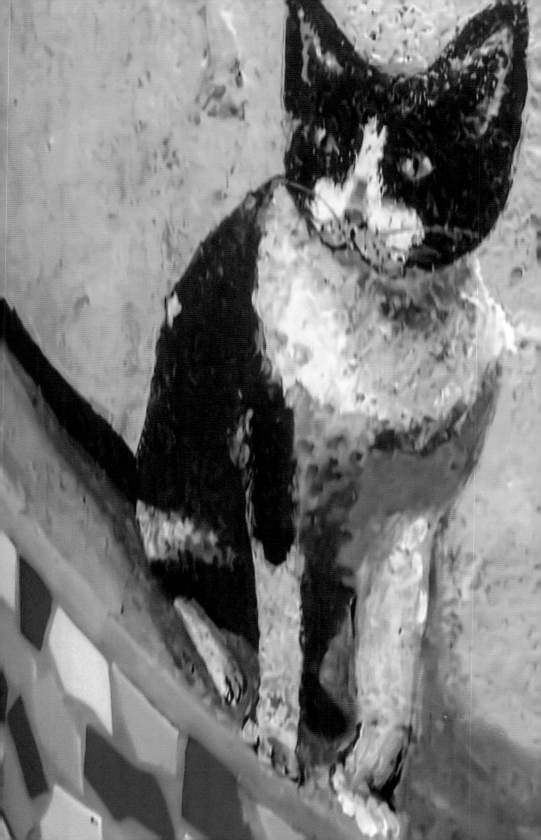

help your pet

Your mom and dad are on Medicare so you don't have to worry about their medical bills.

How about your dog? If you don't like him you'll dump him. Many people do and the pets daily perish in animal shelters, sometimes from starvation.

On top of helping your own pet, you can help other pets, all the animals in fact.

If you are rich, don't care about money and can afford a vet, your pet will still have the nasty side effects from the drugs. They are the same drugs after all.

I wonder what the dog psychiatrists do during therapy?

Healing Animals

Boris the Cat - conjunctivitis healed

Boris the cat had recurring conjunctivitis for years and a few weeks ago it occurred to me that I could help him. On the first occasion I just placed my palms over his eyes for a short while and only managed 20 seconds or so before he wriggled off. Two weeks later I did it again for around a minute, this time more intensely. A few days after that when I saw him again one eye was completely clear and the other was still a bit crusty. On this occasion he was purring as I opened his bio-field and did most of the eye protocol along with positive therapy. Anyway, after just three sessions his eyes are green and glowing and poor old Boris is now one happy cat. :)

My dog saved from kidney failure by Bioenergy Healing

Back in October, our dog, HeyBoy, got really sick – extreme lethargy, vomiting, diarrhea. We made an appointment at the vet but had to wait 3 days. On the night before his appointment, I felt as though he was literally dying. So at midnight, we rushed him to the emergency animal hospital.

His kidney levels were through the roof. He was diagnosed with chronic renal failure. The vet told us he'd be lucky to live a few more months, but most likely (based upon his blood work) it would be a matter of weeks.

I had just returned from level one training in Sarasota and when the doctor left the room, I told my husband that I didn't believe one word of the doctor's prognosis and knew that this condition could be reversed. HeyBoy was put on intravenous fluids and the following morning was transferred to our local vet clinic. He continued his intravenous fluids for the next two days and we brought him home.

Immediately, I started doing Bioenergy healing on him. After the first week, his blood work was redone, and all his levels had dropped into acceptable, although not normal, ranges. We were hopeful but he was still lethargic, had lost 9 pounds, wasn't interested in eating, and still required subcutaneous fluids under the skin daily. I continued Bioenergy after waiting the 7 days. He definitely started feeling better, but was far from being perky and alert. I had to be out of town during the first week of October, so I made arrangements for Zoran to work on him long distance during my absence.

HeyBoy had more blood work done after Zoran's sessions and the blood levels had continued to improve to near normal ranges... And HeyBoy was gaining his weight back. YAY!

He also started getting VERY verbal and his language comprehension increased dramatically. He seemed to already know certain words we didn't even know he knew like "toy" and "bone." And he started to want to play.

Late this afternoon, his blood results came in from the blood that was tested again. ALL blood levels are in the mid-normal range. ALL OF THEM!!!!!!.

His conjunctivitis in his left eye (eye therapy protocol) and his bloody diarrhea (intestinal protocol) and his aggressiveness (psychogenic protocol) had completely cleared up – forgot to mention these issues.

And he is wagging his tail over every little thing.

It's awesome to walk this walk with him.

Dog Tumors Gone using Purebioenergy Healing

In April of 2014 I participated in and hosted on my property a Purebioenergy Healing Group led by a certified therapist. As we gathered, my dog, Kona, was around but not particularly interested in what we were doing, until the therapist began working on the first client. Kona would come up and poke his nose into where her hands were and would not leave her or the person receiving the energy alone. He had to be in the middle of it the whole time, he would just not leave us. We were all amused at how interested he was in what was going on.

Initially I didn't even think about healing for Kona, but since he was all over the therapist and would not leave her alone to do the healings, we began to talk about him and I began to share details about him and his ailments.

"He was covered in tumors, I mean covered."

Kona has been with us since he was born, my oldest son helped deliver him and he was the runt of the litter. He grew to be the largest of all of the pups! He's been such a huge part of our family ever since.

I mentioned to Elizabeth and the group that he was extremely old (much older than a dog of his size and breed typically lives) and suffered from severe arthritis and senility, as well as tumors all over his body. He was covered in tumors, I mean covered. I had counted 11 tumors on him at that time.

I said that we were very worried we were going to lose him because we had noticed a steep decline in his health and mobility, particularly since December of that year when he stopped being able to go up and down the stairs to sleep with us at night, which was traumatic for all of us. He stopped going outside unless prompted by one of us. He stopped jumping up on the couch, he struggled to get up from his doggie bed, and just stopped moving around as much as he could before.

"He was a puppy again."

E. offered to work on Kona while there, so he received therapy beginning the first day. While she worked on him Kona became very still and then laid down on his side and sprawled out on the floor in front of us. It was amazing. He seemed to understand what was going on, and even made movements as if he were trying to communicate with her while she was treating him.

After she worked on him that first day, shortly after E. left, Kona started running around! He ran outside and inside like he was a puppy again, grabbing toys and running back and forth and wanting to play. He was so happy, it was incredible. It was unbelievable. Kona continued to receive therapy with the group each day. On day four right as the therapy was beginning, to our surprise Kona came over and jumped up on the couch to sit with some of the women in the group!

"Where are all of Kona's tumors, did he have surgery?"

I was happy that Kona had regained some of his youthful spirit and that his pain was eased as part of the therapy. I didn't even think to feel his tumors.

About a week later, my oldest son came to visit and immediately went over to hug Kona. I was in the other room when I hear 'Mom, where are all of Kona's tumors, did he have surgery?' I came in the room and he had felt Kona from the tip of his nose all the way down his body. I felt Kona up and down, looked at my son and said 'Oh my God, E. worked on him a week ago. My son looked back at me with tears in his eyes and we both just started crying.

Kona went from having 11 tumors down to only one, that had shrunk to half the size of what it was before.

This testimonial is from Kona's Owner, Tracy Kelly. Kona is 14 years old.

Mr. T's skull alignment

Mr T had a significant blow to the front of his head that shoved his bones up to the left. You can see the dent in the nasal and frontal bones, which impaired his sinuses and the lacrimal bone moved out in front of his left eye, which impaired his vision and blocked his tear duct.

He also was very sedate in his personality, which is strange for him.

…And now, of course, he has cleared his sinuses, can see out of left eye, and is back to his crazy self. It's awesome.

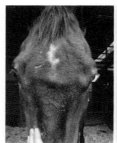 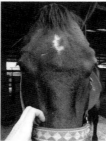 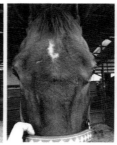 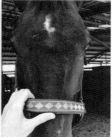

Day 1   *Day 2*   *Day 3*   *Day 4*

Little Miracles At Horseshoe Acres In Boca Raton

Barin is our "good old boy", a 30 year old Guatemalan Hunter, who enjoys his retirement and getting fed copious amounts of carrots from the children at the facility.

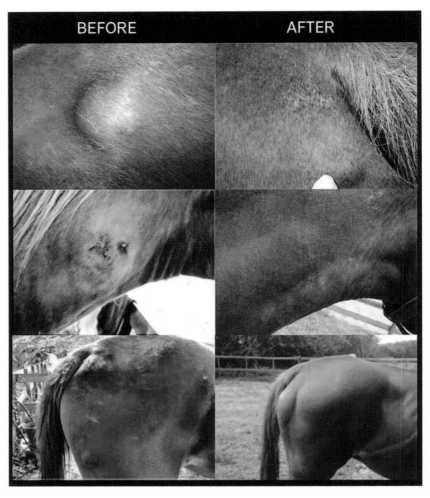

BEFORE AFTER

Barin was rescued by his previous owners from an abusive home. He came to us two years ago in terrible shape. Countless hours of love and care have allowed him to recover and overcome several of his health issues. But as an old horse in his thirties, which in human years is equal to their nineties, he will always remain a skinny, more fragile "boy". Another issue for Barin is that he suffers from an autoimmune disease. He grows big abscesses all over his body which break open and infect themselves over and over again.

We treated his autoimmune disease through cortisone, antibiotic and vet work. We could usually always maintain his condition but during his last outbreak, in April 2013, there seemed to be no healing or relief for Barin. Despite all medications and efforts his body kept on producing abscesses and finally his owners and myself decided that it might be time to give-up.

Just as we had given up hope, one of my client's mother offered her help. A certified Purebioenergy healer took on Barin's case and offered her services. I must admit, even though I'm open-minded and believe in Bioenergy healing I was very skeptical when it came to treating Barin.

Barin seemed to be too weak to have enough healing power in him for the 1 hour long sessions, for 4 consecutive days. But thankfully he and Sabina proved me wrong. After one set of 4 treatment sessions and a boost up by two therapists together (Zoran visited), Barin started to gain back his strength! He stopped producing new abscesses and the old one either disappeared or opened up and healed! The pictures don't really show the magnitude of his healing condition but IT is visible how much his appearance has changed.

Today Barin stills enjoys his life at the pasture and we hope that he will enjoy several more healthy years. Thank you for saving his life! We are grateful for our little miracle at Horseshoe Farms.

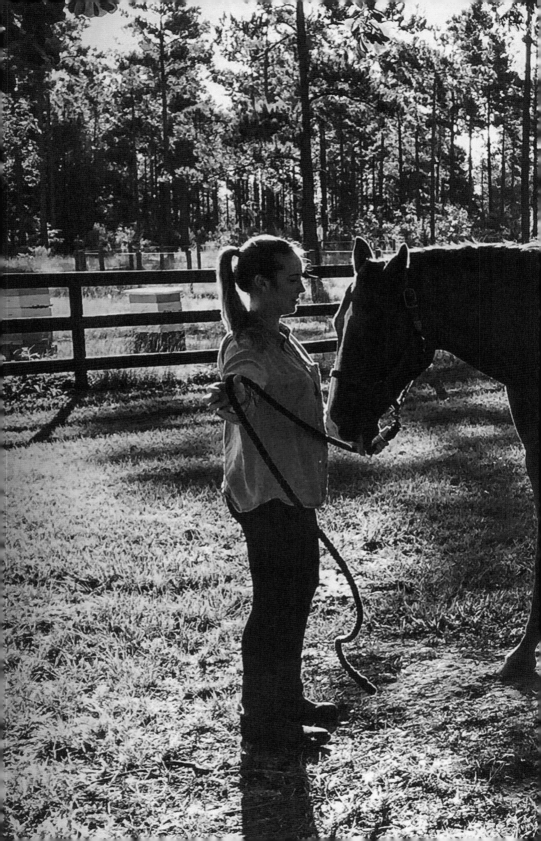

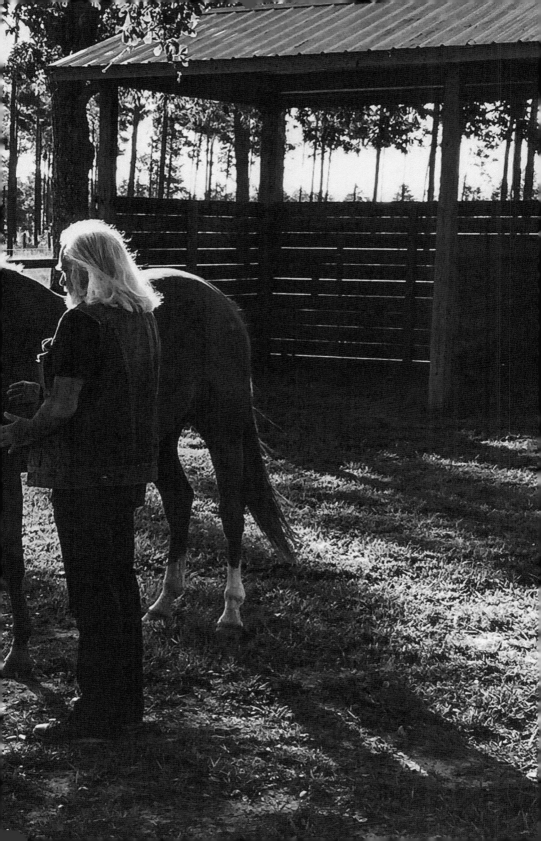

Acknowledgments

I want to thank absolutely everybody that contributed to this book.

We never really counted the testimonials we received over the years. Most of them are not included in this book because they run in hundreds, maybe thousands. I want to thank the *Students and Patients* for those, unpublished stories, as well.

Nothing would have been possible if *Stephanie Coté* didn't collect and archive them.

Then the whole collection of hundreds and hundreds of notes, emails and letters was sent to New Zealand, for *Cathie Lindsey* to sift through it, find the "top stories" and then the "top of the tops".

Thank you *Stephanie* and *Cathie*.

We tried to keep the words the way people wrote them. There are American, British and Canadian spellings. Many of the contributors are not native English speakers and I think it is great that so many people from all these countries around the globe are using Bioenergy.

Thank you *Ivan Pešić*, this book's designer, for a great job and for putting up with me through the working process.

Actually, I want to thank everybody for putting up with me.

Zoran

Disclaimer

Bioenergy Therapy, performed as taught in PUREBIOENERGY® training courses, is a highly effective complementary therapy for promoting health and healing, but it is NOT a replacement for conventional medical treatment.

A PUREBIOENERGY® practitioner does not diagnose illness, disease or any other physical or mental disorder. As such, the PUREBIOENERGY® practitioner does not interfere with medical procedures, prescribed medical treatment or any use of pharmaceuticals, nor do they perform any spinal manipulation.

The information contained in this book and presented in our seminars is for educational purposes only.

63597517R00085

Made in the USA
Lexington, KY
11 May 2017